THE WORLD'S GREATEST DOCTOR

J. EUGENE WILSON, J.D.

ISBN   9780976790310

About the Author:

J. Eugene Wilson, J.D. is an Atlanta attorney who has studied health for over 40 years and is a life member of The National Health Federation. He has written four other books and has practiced law for 54 ½ years. He has a great interest in good health for everyone and believes he had to study about good health as a self-defense measure because we are losing the so-called war against cancer.

He believes that the California doctor he has written about is the World's Greatest because he used a standard treatment for his patients, and 30 days later over 90% of his patients were cured. He used the "Cold Sheet Treatment" for his patients who were dying and succeeded in getting many of them well.

TABLE OF CONTENTS

Notice · · · · · · · · · · · · · · · · · 14

Foreword · · · · · · · · · · · · · · · · 15

Separating the Wheat from the Chaff · · · · · · · · · 18

The World's Greatest Doctor · · · · · · · · · · · 19

Chapter One- Introduction · · · · · · · · · · · · 27

Chapter Two- Cancer · · · · · · · · · · · · · 29

- Chemotherapy & Bone Marrow Transplants · · · · · 31
- Colon Cancer May Be Cured with Ellagimax · · · · 32
- Buying Ellagimax · · · · · · · · · · · · 33
- You May Destroy Breast & Prostate Cancer
- Eliminating Bowel Gas · · · · · · · · · · 35
- Probiotic Treatments for Gas
- Cancer Treatments May Change in Future · · · · · 36
- The Best Treatment

Chapter Three- The Colon · · · · · · · · · · · 37

- How Much Fecal Matter Can a Person Hold? · · · · 40
- A Clean Colon May Help Prevent Cancer
- How Bad Can It Get? My Constipation Record Breakers. 41
- What the Heck is a Normal Poop Anyway? · · · · · 42
- Normal Consistency · · · · · · · · · · · 43
- Signs of Constipation
- Bowel Cleansing Can Be the Cure for Any Digestive
  Disease · · · · · · · · · · · · · · · 44
- Dr. Schulze's Intestinal Detoxification Program · · · **46**

Chapter Four- The Doctor's Greatest Secret · · · · · · 50

- Get Well by Dr. Schulze · · · · · · · · · · **51**

Chapter Five- There Are No Incurable Diseases · · · · · · 59

• Cold Sheet Treatment · · · · · · · · · · · · · · 60

Chapter Six- Overcoming Impotence Naturally· · · · · · · **63**

• Genetics, Natural Healing, and Impotency
• What Causes All Disease? · · · · · · · · · · · · · 65
• The Cure for All Disease · · · · · · · · · · · · · 66
• Maybe, All IS Well? · · · · · · · · · · · · · · · 67
• Is it Really a Disease, or a Blessing from God?
• Potency & Fertility- Survival of the Fittest · · · · · · 68
• Impotency & Fertility- Is it just Bad Luck or Bad Living? 70
• Medical Doctors: Are They Miracle Workers or the Anti-Christ? · · · · · · · · · · · · · · · · · 71
• If God & Nature are Saying No, Then You have to Say Yes · 72
• Diseases of the Male Reproductive System · · · · · · 73
• Erectile Dysfunction · · · · · · · · · · · · · · · 74
• Bad Circulation
• Hormone Imbalance · · · · · · · · · · · · · · · 75
• Prescription and Street Drug Use
• Anatomy & Physiology of the Male Reproductive System · 76
• Diseases of the Female Reproductive System · · · · · 77
• Puberty & Sexual Maturity
• P.M.S., Abnormal Uterine Bleeding & Menstrual Disorders · · · · · · · · · · · · · · · · · · · 80
• P.M.S, It's Very Real
• What Causes P.M.S.? · · · · · · · · · · · · · · · 81
• Symptoms of P.M.S. · · · · · · · · · · · · · · · 82
• The Natural Solution to P.M.S., Non-Medicated Awareness · · · · · · · · · · · · · · · · · · · 83
• Herbal Medication for P.M.S. · · · · · · · · · · · 85
• Abnormal Menstrual Pain & Bleeding · · · · · · · · 86

- Hormonal Imbalance· · · · · · · · · · · · · · 87
- Constipation & Toxicity · · · · · · · · · · · 88
- Pelvic Inflammatory Disease · · · · · · · · · 89
- Dr. Schulze's Herbal Feminine Douche Recipe

Chapter Seven- How To Improve the Quality of Your Life · · 91

- The Law of Diminishing Returns
- Just Say No to Drugs! · · · · · · · · · · · · 92
- Am I Too Aggressive? · · · · · · · · · · · 94
- What Do Pain Relief, Liver Death and the Movie 'The Fugitive' All Have In Common? · · · · · · · · · 95
- Sudden Liver Cell Death!
- The Liver · · · · · · · · · · · · · · · · · 96
- Energy & Nutrition
- Detoxification · · · · · · · · · · · · · · · 97
- Now for the Number Freaks· · · · · · · · · · 98
- When Your Liver Gets Sick · · · · · · · · · 99
- Intra Hepatic Jaundice· · · · · · · · · · · · 100
- Viral Hepatitis
- Extra Hepatic Jaundice
- The Gallbladder · · · · · · · · · · · · · · 101
- The Liver Flush & What It Does · · · · · · · 102

Chapter Eight- There IS a Cure for the Common Cold · · · 103

Chapter Nine- What About Success Stories? · · · · · · 116

- I Broke My Own Rules· · · · · · · · · · · · **118**
- Cancer, Cancer · · · · · · · · · · · · · · **120**

Chapter Ten- Patient & Customer Success Stories· · · · · **123**

- Jim's Interview · · · · · · · · · · · · · · **129**
- Toni's Letter · · · · · · · · · · · · · · · **134**
- Hilda's Interview · · · · · · · · · · · · · **135**
- Email from Dave B · · · · · · · · · · · · **143**

- Cold Sheet Treatment Success Stories · · · · · · · **144**

Chapter Eleven- To Your Good Health · · · · · · · · **146**

- Chemotherapy & Lung Cancer · · · · · · · · · · 148
- Food May Cure Your Cancer · · · · · · · · · · 149
- How to Use Asparagus · · · · · · · · · · · · 150
- Fish Oil · · · · · · · · · · · · · · · · 151
- Rheumatoid Arthritis · · · · · · · · · · · · 153
- Migraines
- Lupus · · · · · · · · · · · · · · · · · 154
- Other Ailments Helped by Fish Oil
- Preventing Cancer · · · · · · · · · · · · · · 155
- Cherries
- High Blood Pressure
- Fava Beans
- Flu Shots May be Dangerous · · · · · · · · · · 156

Chapter Twelve- Some Good Ideas · · · · · · · · · 158

- Apple Cider Vinegar
- Garlic · · · · · · · · · · · · · · · · · 160
- Flax Seed Oil + Low Fat Cottage Cheese · · · · · · 161
- Alzheimer's Disease · · · · · · · · · · · · · **163**
- Gout · · · · · · · · · · · · · · · · · 164
- Carrots
- Headaches
- Pain In Lumbar Vertebrae, Sacrum & Sciatic Nerve · · 166
- How You May Stop Losing Your Hair · · · · · · · **168**

Chapter Thirteen- Garlic & Other Cures · · · · · · · **169**

- Garlic May Cure Your Cancer
- The Salt Treatment May Cure Your Cancer · · · · · 170
- How to Take the Salt Water Treatment · · · · · · · 174
- How to Use Salt Water for Cleansing · · · · · · · 175
- How You May Add Years to Your Life · · · · · · · 177

- Migraine Headaches · · · · · · · · · · · · · · 178
- Only 30 Days to Live · · · · · · · · · · · · · 179
- Melanoma
- What Causes Arthritis? · · · · · · · · · · · · 180
- Back to my Friend with Melanoma · · · · · · · · 181
- Why Did He Get Cancer?
- Indium- The Missing Trace Mineral
- Cayenne May Cure You · · · · · · · · · · · · · · 183
- Cayenne Is Great for Stopping Bleeding · · · · · · 184
- Cayenne May Save You if You Have a Heart Attack
- Cayenne May Get Rid of Your High Blood Pressure· · 185
- Cayenne May Heal Your Brain Cancer Also
- L-Arginine (see page 186 also) · · · · · · · · · 185

Chapter Fourteen- Non-Toxic Therapies & Diagnostic Tests · 187

Directory (see page 193)

Chapter Fifteen- Dr. Clark · · · · · · · · · · · · 200

Chapter Sixteen- Vitamin Q · · · · · · · · · · · · 204

- Cancer Treatments
- Only 25% of Cancer Victims Die of Cancer · · · · 205
- Getting CoQ10
- Treatment Results · · · · · · · · · · · · · · 206
- Another Good Vitamin Q to Take · · · · · · · · 208
- Another Very Absorbable Form · · · · · · · · · 209
- What is L-Carnitine?
- What Does L-Carnitine Do That Is So Important?
- Is There Another Fuel That Your Heart Needs? · · · 210
- What Are the Benefits of Taking Them Together?
- Warning: Beware of MIG Blasts · · · · · · · · 211
- Other Diseases · · · · · · · · · · · · · · · 212
- Heart Disease
- Ideas You May Use · · · · · · · · · · · · · · 214

- Liver Kampo

Chapter Seventeen- Spectro Chrome · · · · · · · · · · 216

Chapter Eighteen- Royal Rife· · · · · · · · · · · · **269**

- Results of Rife Treatments
- A Great Discovery · · · · · · · · · · · · · · · 271
- Sick People Have Very Poor Immune Systems
- My Experience with Rife's Machine · · · · · · · 272
- Kill the Viruses by Shocking Them to Death

Chapter Nineteen- Some Ideas You May Have Missed · · · 274

- New Miracle Prostate Cancer Treatment · · · · · · 276
- New Hope for Colon Cancer · · · · · · · · · · · 278
- Vitamin D Connection
- Oral Urea for Living Cancer · · · · · · · · · · 279
- Raw Thyroid, Raw Thymus, etc. · · · · · · · · · 280
- Glutathione · · · · · · · · · · · · · · · · · 282
- Anti-Cancer Strategies · · · · · · · · · · · · 282
- More About Parkinson's· · · · · · · · · · · · 284
- How You May Reduce Your High Blood Pressure · · 285
- Some Anti-Oxidants You May Take · · · · · · · · 286
- Still More About Parkinson's

Chapter Twenty- Anthrax· · · · · · · · · · · · · · · 287

- Colloidal Silver (CS) · · · · · · · · · · · · · 289
- Living Essential Oils · · · · · · · · · · · · · 291
- Lavender · · · · · · · · · · · · · · · · · · 292
- Oregano
- Theives
- Why We Should Use Essential Oils Instead of Herbs? · 293
- Eucalyptus Oil
- Let's Keep Things In Perspective · · · · · · · · 294

Chapter Twenty One- DMSO · · · · · · · · · · · · · 296

Chapter Twenty Two- The Ultimate Healer · · · · · · · 300

- Only God Can Heal You · · · · · · · · · · · · · 301
- Another Idea for Healing · · · · · · · · · · · 302
- Lorraine Day, M.D. · · · · · · · · · · · · · · 303

Chapter Twenty Three- How to Add Ten to Fifteen Years
or More to Your Life · · · · · · · · · · · · · · · 306

- Get Rid of Your Amalgam Fillings Now!
- Eliminate All Sodium Fluoride from Your Consumption 307
- Cleanse Yourself Internally to Remove Toxins
- Enjoy a Good Juice Fast Twice a Year · · · · · · · 308
- Cleanse Your Liver & Kidneys
- Get Exercise & Sunshine Daily · · · · · · · · · 309
- Avoid Taking Drugs If Possible
- Buy Your Drugs from Canada to Save Money
- Don't Smoke & Avoid Second-Hand Smoke · · · · · 310
- Eliminate of Reduce the Sweets in Your Diet · · · · 311
- Reduce or Eliminate Alcohol from Your Diet
- Eliminate Aluminum from Your Diet · · · · · · · 313
- Avoid Taking Aspirin to Thin Your Blood
- Eliminate Stress from Your Life
- EDTA Chelation Therapy with Suppositories · · · · 315
- Your Immune System
- Rebuild Your Immune system · · · · · · · · · · 317
- Homocysteine · · · · · · · · · · · · · · · · 318

THE WORLD'S GREATEST DOCTOR

NOTICE

The information in this book is, for the most part, based upon my personal experiences, and my knowledge learned from studying health information for the last 40 years. We know that each person is different and each situation is unique, so the author and publisher urges the readers of this book to check with a well qualified professional before using any procedure if there is any question concerning appropriateness.

Because there is always some risk involved, the author and publisher are not responsible for any consequences or adverse effects resulting from the use of any procedures, preparations or suggestions described in this book. If you are not willing to assume the risk, please do not use the book. You should feel free to consult with a well qualified health professional or physician, as this is a sign of great wisdom to seek a second or third opinion.

WARNING: The statements made in this book have NOT been evaluated or approved by the F.D.A. We must also legally warn you that even though your medical doctor has had absolutely no training in Herbology or Natural Healing, if you are ill, have any disease or are pregnant or nursing, to consult your medical doctor before attempting any natural or herbal program.

FOREWARD

A number of years ago, John Wayne was talking on his phone with Nat King Cole, a great black singer, who was suffering with terminal cancer. Mr. Wayne tried to cheer him up and here is what he said:

"I LICKED CANCER - SO CAN YOU!" Unfortunately he was wrong insofar as Nat King Cole was concerned for he died of cancer soon thereafter.

After learning more about John Wayne, I came to the conclusion that he was wrong also when he said he licked cancer. He didn't win the battle against cancer at all, because he had cancer when he died.

When John Wayne got his first cancer, it was lung cancer, apparently because of his smoking so much. He had his first operation for cancer in 1964 and returned home soon thereafter. Sometime later, he was in the hospital again for his second cancer operation, which was for stomach cancer. He returned again much later for his third operation, which was for cancer of the bowel. This was his final operation for cancer, which was shortly before his death in 1979. Dr. Bernard Jensen, one of the all time great doctors, who died at age 92 during June of 2001, was of the opinion that Mr. Wayne's bowel should have been checked very carefully at the earliest sign of cancer of his lungs. He says in his book DR JENSEN'S GUIDE TO BETTER BOWEL CARE, "since… the condition of the bowel is related to conditions in all the other parts of the body, we should look to the bowel first, not last. I'm as sure as I can be from my experience with so many others that there was bowel trouble in John Wayne's case a long time before there was any problem in his stomach or his lungs. IF HIS BOWEL HAD BEEN TAKEN CARE OF EARLIER, PROBLEMS MIGHT NOT HAVE OCCURRED ELSEWHERE. …If we learn to care for the bowel, we can avoid the many conditions associated with a toxic colon."

It is always so unfortunate when any of us dies of cancer, since it seems so unnecessary. I believe that if we educate ourselves and learn how to avoid getting cancer as well as how to get well when we do have cancer, we will be the winners and not the losers to cancer. Since cancer is caused by parasites plus pollution, it would seem that we should be intelligent enough to win the battle by destroying the parasites, as well as eliminating the pollution they depend upon, or both, and become totally free of cancer. Developing the necessary knowledge to win this contest is merely self defense. The purpose of this book is to give sufficient information so that we may be able to protect ourselves from getting cancer as well as getting well if we do have cancer. We know that the medical association still uses the cut, burn and poison treatments which were developed about 60 years ago. We also know that they still do not work very well and that more people than ever are still dying of cancer. If you do not believe this, please read the obituary in your newspaper and contact some of the families who lost a loved one due to cancer, and find out if they didn't die even though they obtained medical treatment. We know that of all the people who get cancer, about 50% of them will die from some form of heart problem, and about 25% will die from some other cause. The other 25% will die from the cancer. We know that many of those who die from some other cause died from the treatment the doctor inflicted upon them.

Since drugs are poisonous, we know that some are more poisonous than others. Chemotherapy is apparently a very poisonous drug since so many people die from overdoses. Since we are all different, the doctors don't know how much chemotherapy any of us can withstand before it kills us. Many times I've read in the obituary of the local newspaper that someone died from a chemotherapy overdose. This probably happens much more than we realize. I even read of one young man who had 6 very good friends, and, to his utter amazement, all 6 of them were told by their doctor that they had developed cancer during the same year, and all 6 died from overdoses of chemotherapy. They were apparently all using the same doctor and the doctor may have given the same dosage to each. I presume they each only took what the doctor ordered, and then died. How could this be allowed to happen? None of them had cancer and all died because they were poisoned to death.

We know that back in 1900, there were few people coming down with cancer. One report claims that only about 1 in 25 people developed cancer in their bodies then, whereas today 1 in every 3 females and 50% of all males will end up with cancer during their lifetimes. This is increasing in epidemic proportions and may reach 60% soon. This is not what I would call winning the war against cancer, but just the opposite. One way to look at it is to simply say that the alleged wars against cancer are nothing more than phony wars. This sounds to me like a scheme for the doctors to make more money from us. What do you think?

NOTE: A number of chapters of this book contain quotations of Dr. Richard Schulze, but sometimes the author has changed the wording to improve the grammar. Dr. Schulze is an outstanding doctor and has accomplished great things in treating his patients as you will see. He also has excelled in saving patients lives who came to him on their way to the cemetery, because he used such great treatments on them, which is discussed in Chapters 4 and 10 of this book. Hopefully some of you may find this information interesting and educational. If you need medical treatments, the author recommends that you obtain the services of a very competent medical doctor. See Chapter 14 for a list of excellent medical doctors for treatments of cancer.

May this book give you a better insight into some of the best treatments for cancer and their results. Hopefully it will start you in the right direction for valid and successful treatments of your cancer.

SEPARATING THE WHEAT FROM THE CHAFF

This is important as you will read lots of invalid, and incorrect information telling you what to do for a given ailment. Sometimes you will read that you should only take so much of a vitamin or mineral and the amount is what you need for survival, and not for good health. Most times the amount listed is much too low, but sometimes it is much too high. One doctor who is very smart and normally gives very good advice indicated that you should take 1200 milligrams of magnesium and stated that this was a very small amount. I know of my own knowledge that he is excessively high. I tried taking 500 mg for some time and found this amount to be too much for me. I believe everyone should take a calcium magnesium capsule each night shortly before bed, and I believe a combination capsule of 500 mg of calcium and 250 mg of magnesium is sufficient. This may help us to avoid heart problems. The doctor probably meant 120 mg and 1200 was simply a misprint.

We know that a number of vegetables we eat contains magnesium and if we eat lots of vegetables such as spinach, turnip greens, collard greens and other such vegetables, we will get much of the magnesium we need and when we add the amount we take just before bedtime, we may have more than we need as I did when I was taking 500 mg of magnesium and 500 mg of calcium. Too much is worse than not enough, so I learned from experience that I did not need to take it every night. When I do take it at night, I only take 250 mg of magnesium and 500 mg of calcium. Pay attention to your body. It knows what you need and what is best for you.

THE WORLD'S GREATEST DOCTOR

Chapters 3 through 12 of this book, for the most part, pertain to THE WORLD'S GREATEST DOCTOR. And the other 13 chapters contain OTHER INFORMATION. If you are ill with cancer or some other severe disease or sickness, you may wish to turn to and read Chapters 4 and 10 for some excellent information you may use to treat your illness. You may want to place an order with the American Botanical Pharmacy for some drugless materials you will use to cure your illness. If you are dying or seriously ill with cancer of some other ailment, you will undoubtedly wish to go on The Incurables Program so you will have a good chance of recovering, that is, if you have a sufficient time left to receive meaningful treatments. "The Cold Sheet Treatment" is beneficial if you are seriously ill or dying.

In a newsletter dating back to 1999, Dr. Shulze says that there is nothing more dangerous and politically incorrect these days than to dare say that there is a cure for cancer. So he says it, "There is a cure for cancer, but not with Medical Doctors, Hospitals, Drugs or even Alternative Programs."

Medicine can't find a cure because they are looking for a pill or a chemical that will kill cancer cells without killing the rest of you, and to do this while you still live a cancer-causing lifestyle. While their egos keep them in search for the impossible, they build hospital cancer wings with donations from junk food hamburger chains.

Government can't help us because politicians took their campaign money from the industries that pollute our air, water, food and earth with cancer-causing chemicals. They will not bite the hand that feeds them.

And if you are waiting for a cure from the multi-billion dollar cancer research hospitals and institutes, you are in real trouble. Oh, they know what causes cancer, but you will never hear it because their funding comes from the tobacco and other industries that cause cancer. They also know cancer cures, but you'll never hear about any of them. Do you really, honestly expect them to commit financial suicide and put hundreds of thousands of people out of work?

And if you're hoping for a cure with Alternative Medicine, you're in for a big disappointment. It won't kill you like the medical treatment, but today's gutless practitioners use wimpy dosages and ineffective, lightweight programs. They'll heal your dry skin and bad breath, so you'll still die but you'll look and smell good.

The bottom line is, if you have cancer, your only hope is to heal yourself. Over the last 20 years I have had thousands of patients in my clinic and other clinics all over the world following my protocols that did heal themselves of cancer.

Medicine has lost the war against cancer. At the turn of the century, only 1 out of 25 people got cancer. Today it is 1 out of 3, a fraction away from 1 out of 2.

Why are more people getting cancer today than ever before in history?

Why has the Medical and Government "War on Cancer" been lost?

Why, with all of our money, modern technology and research, can't we find a cure?

Why can't we find a drug to stop this plague?

The answer to all of these questions is very simple. There is no magic bullet cure for cancer and there never will be.

WARNING: The following opinion on cancer by Dr. Shultze is based on 20 years of clinical practice and observation, but is extremely controversial. We are forced to tell you that it is printed under the First Amendment of the United States Constitution, which grants us the right to discuss openly and freely all matters of public concern, and to express viewpoints no matter how controversial or unaccepted they may be. We are also forced to tell you that if you are sick, ill or have any disease to see a medical doctor immediately.

For the last 100 years medicine has been looking for and hoping to find a chemical and surgical cure for cancer. The same as Ponce de Leon searched for the Fountain of Youth, but never found it. The same as the Alchemists tried to turn lead into gold, but never could. Medicine searched for a chemical cure for cancer and ignored lifestyle, prevention, diet and detoxification programs. Medicine has totally failed to find their magic bullet for cancer, and for every other major disease from arthritis to diabetes. In fact, many scientists and medical statisticians claim that most magic bullets used to date have probably killed more patients than the cancer did. Most agree that the magic bullets, especially chemotherapy, killed the patient much quicker.

It sounded too good to be true, and it was. At the turn of the century, medicine rose to power by selling a myth, by telling people that they could live with no self control, no responsibility, burn the candle at both ends, live life in the fast lane and when you finally got ill, they could fix you with a pill.

Modern Medicine actually thought they could ignore Mother Nature and spit in the face of God. They tried to create a system of healing where the patient did not have to take any responsibility for themselves. Doctors hoped in the future that a person could ignore all the laws of science, nature and God. They hoped that you could live a life of decadence, eat anything, drink anything, do anything and think anything, and they could fix any problem with a drug, a magic bullet.

This idea sold a lot of people, why not, a life full of smoking, drinking, drugs, eating garbage food, and no spiritual practice- one big decadent party. This caused the tobacco, liquor, junk food and pharmaceutical industries to skyrocket, and in turn, they supported medicine back and paid for research, hospital wings and medical colleges. Today, we have cancer hospitals built by hamburger chains and tobacco industries funding lung cancer research.

Finally, America and the world is now waking up and realizing the folly of the magic bullet theory and people worldwide are returning to a common sense natural healing lifestyle.

SO THE MEDICAL TREATMENT DOESN'T EVEN WORK, AND WORSE, IT KILLS YOU QUICKER

At a recent symposium on AIDS I attended in Europe, doctors wondered why people in America with AIDS were dying FASTER and from totally different bizarre symptoms and rare diseases than they were in the rest of the world. This international team of expert medical doctors and top immunologists agreed that in America, AIDS patients are not actually dying from the disease, but from the side effects of the medical treatment, especially the drugs. In my clinic I discovered a similar but startling fact on the survival rates of my patients who had cancer. The ones that did nothing, just let the cancer spread and eventually died, well most of them outlived the patients that underwent aggressive medical cancer therapy. They not only had a longer life, but also a much better quality of life. It seems as though the medical treatment of cancer is hazardous to your health and definitely kills you quicker than the disease.

On the other hand, my patients who decided to stop doing the things that caused their cancer in the first place and started following programs that are known to prevent and even heal cancer, well, they far outlived all the life-span estimates for cancer patients, outlived their oncologists, and in fact, most of them are still alive today.

I spent the last 10 years of my clinical practice helping people who were dying from degenerative diseases, killer diseases, and supposedly incurable diseases. I learned that there are a lot of natural healing routines, herbal formulae, health books and healing hypothesis that are effective for pimples and dandruff, but they are useless for killer diseases. My patients followed these programs and got sicker. The reason my patients were able to heal their so-called incurable diseases, the reason my patients created healing miracles is because I didn't stop kicking their asses until they were well.

Natural and Alternative doctors fool around balancing your aura and spritzing you with essential oils. What I call finishing treatments. Even if they get tough, they still use wimpy programs with impotent pathetic dosages. At least a medical doctor knows how to treat killer diseases with intensity- they will cut the top of your head off and carve a tumor out, or cut your testicles off or your ovaries out. Get it? If you are going to heal yourself of a killer disease with natural healing instead of modern medicine, you have got to pull out all the stops, turn the intensity up to 110%, put the pedal to the metal and don't look back.

I have never killed any of my patients. No, I never killed one, but I pushed the limits and took my methods to the MAX. I may have turned some of my patients inside out with wheat-grass juice or the cold sheet treatment, but I never killed, or even hurt, one of them. I could never put too much ice in the ice bath or push them too hard in their emotional healing. I never gave them too much cayenne pepper, purged them too much, cleansed them too much or had one die from a vegetable juice overdose. I tried, but they didn't break. I dared some of them to go ahead and die on me, but they didn't. THEY LIVED, THRIVED AND CELEBRATED LONG, HEALTHY, VITAL, HAPPY LIVES. THEY HEALED THEMSELVES!

No one is dying from over zealous natural doctors, over intense programs and overdoses of herbs. They are dying from not enough!

When I visit my students' clinics in America, Europe, or anywhere in the world, often they line up their worst cases for me in the hallway. These were the patients they hadn't been able to get well. Patients that were not responding. 99% of the time my student doctors are doing all of the right things, just not enough of them and not often enough. TURN UP THE INTENSITY.

The big problem is that most natural doctors are afraid of hurting someone. They didn't want to break the patient or push them too far. If a patient has a terminal, incurable or killer disease, TURN UP THE INTENSITY, TRY TO KILL THEM WITH CARROT JUICE, ENEMAS, HERBAL PURGES AND POSITIVE THINKING- YOU

CAN'T. I would scream at these doctors, "What are you afraid of, killing them? They are already dying. You have nothing to lose."

Often I would take what the doctor had the patient doing in one day and I would make them do it in an hour, and then repeat it 8 or 10 more times that day. Push it to the MAX.

People are much tougher than you think. When I looked into the lives of these supposedly frail patients, the way they lived and took care of themselves before they got sick, it was very intense. These people were drinking pints of wrong beverages, smoking cigarettes, and on a steady diet of animal foods and bad attitudes. They never questioned all the ways they tried to kill themselves. They never questioned when they opened their seventh beer why beer comes in six-packs and maybe seven is an overdose. They just chugged it down.

They never questioned that one bag of greasy potato chips or junk snacks was a dosage when they ripped open the next bag, munched it down and changed the tv channel. They didn't call the manufacturer to see if maybe they were overdoing it. They just partied hearty.

Cigarettes, Booze, Sugar, Chocolate, Fast Food, Recreational Drugs, Prescription Drugs, Artificial Everything, Household Toxins, Environmental Pollutants, Bad Relationships and Filling Our Minds with Garbage, WE NEVER QUESTIONED IT, WE NEVER SLOWED IT DOWN, WE NEVER WORRIED ABOUT OVERDOSE. BUT NOW, in healing ourselves, we are concerned about taking an overdose of herbs. We are worried that one too many cups of ginger-root tea and the cold sheet treatment will be too rough. GIVE ME A BREAK!

If people had half the determination, energy and intensity healing themselves and they used partying, tearing themselves down and trying to kill themselves, they could have a healing miracle, ALMOST IMMEDIATELY.

What cured cancer and killer diseases in my clinic? I wish I could give you the detailed answers here and now, but I can't. This is NOT a teaser or a sales pitch for another product. That is not the way I operate or do business. I always skirt, if not break, the law to give you the best healing information I have. I give you more than I legally should. I can't tell you any specific programs for cancer in this forum. If I do, it's simple; I go to jail, and jail doesn't have vegetarian entrees.

If you want my entire program, you have to call my school, toll free at 1-877- TEACH-ME (832-2463) and ask them for my Healing Cancer Naturally audio tape set including my new book, There Are NO Incurable Diseases; Dr. Schulze's Intensive 30 Day Cleansing and Detoxification Program.

Chapter One

Introduction

So, you've got cancer! You are about to make the most important decision of your life. You are preparing to decide what type of treatment you will take to cure your cancer. If you make the wrong decision, you may end up losing your life. If your decision is correct, you may get well and live a long, happy life. The choice is up to you.

THE WORLD'S GREATEST DOCTOR CURED TENS OF THOUSANDS OF CANCER CASES!

This book contains information from the world's greatest doctor telling you his treatments which have saved many thousands of cancer and other patients. Most doctors use the horse and buggy treatment, which has been around for over 60 years, and has never proved to be very effective. The chemotherapy and radiation treatments they give are rated only 1% effective. Since there are treatments which are rated 100% effective, you surely would rather choose the most effective treatments you can get because THIS IS YOUR LIFE WE ARE TALKING ABOUT. Many treatments are listed in this book, and some of them are rated 100% effective. What is so good about this is the fact that you may take more than one treatment at a time, which is rated at 100% effective.

The world's greatest doctor closed his clinic after a number of years of successful cancer and other disease treatments. He soon reopened and then he only took patients who were dying and on their way to the cemetery, AND HE PROCEEDED TO HEAL MANY OF THEM! This book lists the items he used for successfully treating patients for cancer, heart troubles, strokes, headaches, and many other diseases. His results were spectacular. It also lists the items he used for treating those who were dying and had been told by their doctors that there was nothing that could possibly be done to save them. HE EVEN CLAIMS THAT THERE ARE NO INCURABLE DISEASES! He never used drugs to treat his patients and even claims that "you cannot poison yourself well!" He states that doctors try to kill the cancer in their patient's bodies by poisoning them with drugs, and this does not work. This poisons the patients and sometimes they die from an overdose of the poisonous drugs.

Chapter Two

Cancer

Cancer is defined in Dorland's Medical Dictionary as "a malignant tumor."

Research by numerous worldwide researchers tell us that microbes are the culprits. They initiate degeneration of the blood, organs, digestion and our immune systems. As their numbers increase in the billions, the degeneration likewise increases. These microbes then concentrate in our tumors or in our blood, or both. Actually, by the time a tumor develops, degeneration is well established. Many researchers have reached the conclusion that cancer begins with a microbe.

You're probably wondering if the idea that cancer is caused by a microbe, then why do so many doctors day, "We don't know what causes cancer?" One question many may ask is, "Does the definition of cancer as 'cells gone wild' preclude microbes?" We've had information like this kicking around for over 90 years and we've also had the American Cancer Society around for over 90 years. Why haven't they come up with a cure in 90 years? Are they really looking for a cure and never finding it?

The current thinking in the medical field about cancer is to equate tumor with cancer. With this idea, they concentrate on tumor removal by cutting it, burning it or poisoning it. The cancer microbes arise from within. Inasmuch as we are born with them, they are not recognized as foreign and they haven't invaded us. We are their hosts, and when the hosts are healthy, the microbes live in a congenial relationship, and a friendly form. So long as the host nourishes his body with nutrients compatible with health, the microbe remain friendly. Unfortunately, when the hosts receive inadequate nourishment for a prolonged period, these healthy forms of the microbes associated with cancer turn into virulent, antisocial forms, consuming the unhealthy cells and excreting toxins into our bodies.

Under a darkfield microscope, these microbes can be seen in abundance, untouched, in the cancer patient's blood, sparkling like ten thousand lightning bugs in the twilight zone. These microbes exude a hormone and with a darkfield microscope their forms can be seen after they have gained a foothold subsequent to degeneration. By testing for this hormone, Chorionic Gonadotropin (CG), earlier detection is possible. By using a darkfield microscope examination of the patient's blood, if strange creatures are there and if the test for CG is positive, then you know degeneration is under way.

To begin to control cancer, and to head off degeneration long before there is any sign on tumor, it is necessary to use valid and reliable earlier detection tests. To use detection tests earlier, in the belief that a tumor has to be detected first, and that you are willing to wait and watch until a tumor appears, is a myth slated for total destruction. When we believe that cancer is not cancer without a tumor, this precedes acceptance of these earlier tests of impending degeneration and must go. Can you imagine being diagnosed with cancer with earlier detection tests, when there is no tumor? It would be a nightmare for a surgeon to operate with an x-ray showing a location with no tumor. With no tumor, the surgeon will have nothing to shrink with radiation or chemotherapy. We already know that the cut, burn and poison system does not defeat cancer and such mutilation does not remove the microbes out of the patient's system. Numerous swarms of them can be seen in the blood of a patient who has had the treatments using a darkfield microscope.

Chorionic Gonadotropin (CG) can be detected in the urine of the patient long before any tumor can be seen. Control comes from knowing the idiosyncracies of cancer and then outwitting them. Microbiologists have developed a great respect for the cancer microbe's adaptability, its life, excretions and intelligence. They have learned that they are so tough that you can't destroy them short of boiling them, and even this doesn't always work. We recently read where antibiotics had little effect on the microbes as new generations appear tougher than ever. Behring learned that there is no need to poison them as this only kills the host.

Millions of people are being sacrificed like guinea pigs. Although some oncologists are willing to admit their errors, they are not willing to cease and desist the sacrifice of millions of lives and billions of dollars until a humane solution is discovered. Mutilation of the patients continues while the microbes of cancer continues unscathed, and with a darkfield microscope, we can see their activities. When the host's internal body becomes hostile to the microbes, a healthy, harmonious relationship can no longer continue, and the microbes will then revert to the more primitive, fungal state of their ancestors. They then start using blood sugar and unhealthy cells for their food.

The question arises "How does conventional medicine's treatments of cancer stack up against this field of natural, non-toxic, alternative and complementary treatments?" The answer is this, "It is so far behind that it is fading in the distance."

CHEMOTHERAPY & BONE MARROW TRANSPLANTS

In a report in the San Jose Mercury News, Friday, April 16, 1999, they reported that for the past decade, thousands of women with advanced breast cancer have undergone near fatal doses of chemotherapy and bone marrow transplants hoping the experimental therapy would prolong their lives. The first studies on this procedure show that it did not. Stadmauer's study of 553 women with metastatic disease spread to distant organs showed no difference in overall survival between women who had the transplant and women who received standard chemotherapy.

The studies are clearly a disappointment. The cancer researchers had hoped that high dose chemotherapy would be a breakthrough in a disease that kills 43,000 women a year in the United States. Doctors always hope they will be able to give a patient the maximum chemotherapy dose and yet not kill the patient. Unfortunately, we all are different and some people can take more poison than others without dying from the overdose. Since we know that many are killed by taking the poison chemotherapy, I prefer to steer clear of this and to take alternative treatments.

COLON CANCER MAY BE CURED WITH ELLAGIMAX

If you have colon cancer, you may be able to cure it with Ellagimax, a red raspberry product. Here is a testimonial from a patient: "My name is John and during August 2000, I began having severe discomfort in my lower bowel and suspected a recurrance of colon problems for which I had previously had surgery. I went to my doctor and he confirmed that I had several growths, and he immediately took biopsys on each of them. The results showed that two of them were malignant, so the doctor scheduled surgery.

Before the surgery date, I ran into an old friend who told me about the new red raspberry product called Ellagimax. We listened to several testimonials by cancer patients who claimed to have been cured using this treatment, so I decided to try this method before the surgery, because it might work. In just a few days, I agreed with the testimonials because I could tell a difference in the pain and in the size of the growths.

One month after I started the treatments, I notified my friend that all of my cancerous growths were gone, and I had no pain at all. My doctor had already confirmed to me that the growths were gone, and he agreed that I no longer needed surgery since the cancer was all gone.

BUYING ELLAGIMAX

You may buyEllagimax from Advantage Nutraceutuicals by calling this phone number: 800-867-1891 and tell them J. Eugene Wilson referred you to them. The cost for a bottle of 120 Ellagimax is $34.00. A bottle of 120 should last you 20 days, so you may want to order more than one bottle.

YOU MAY DESTROY
BREAST & PROSTATE CANCER

A lady named Mary suffered with some of the classic symptoms of breast cancer such as fatigue, lower back pain, exhaustion, excessive hair loss, and a drastic change in the shape of her breast. She did not know it, but she actually had advanced cancer of her breast. Like most people, she at first didn't believe she had cancer, but she finally accepted this as a fact since she had so many of the symptoms. With all of the suffering she went through, she then just knew she was dying of cancer. The tissue of her breast with cancer was calcifying, so she took a biopsy and this confirmed the cancer.

Mary was fortunate because she went to see a physician who did not want her to submit to the standard cut, burn and poison treatment, which are usually ineffective in producing a cure. She went to a Dr. Garcia, who has successfully used a cancer treatment called INSULIN POTENTIATION THERAPY (IPT) for close to 20 years. In the 1920's, a doctor named Dr. Perex read about insulin being used to treat non-diabetic malnutrition, and decided to use it on himself because he was suffering with a chronic gastrointestinal condition, so he tried this and effectively treated his condition.

When he used IPT on cancer, the results were astonishing. Other doctors started using it and got great results in using it on children with polio paralysis. The doctors learned that cancer needs glucose for energy and are virtually 100% dependent on glucose as their energy source. Because cancer cells are almost totally dependent on glucose, these cells have many, many insulin receptors on their membranes, and this is the way that cancer cells consume glucose. The cancer cells have up to 15 times as many insulin receptors as other normal cells, so they have a great advantage in obtaining glucose when competing with other cells.

Insulin, in addition to opening up cells for glucose to enter, also makes the cell membranes more permeable to other substances, INCLUDIG CHEMOTHERAPY DRUGS. This fact allows doctors to selectively target the cancer drugs to the cancer cells without destroying the other cells. In other words, more chemotherapy will enter the cancer cells in the presence of the insulin. In effect, this causes the chemotherapy drug to kill the cancer cells at 10,000 times the normal rate. This also means that a much smaller dose of chemotherapy can be given each time the treatment is necessary, and the chemotherapy is not so devastating on the patient.

The doctor told Mary that she would probably need between 12 and 20 treatments. He also stated they would soon know if the treatments were effective.

Mary had her first treatment and said it seemed to help and she did feel better afterwards. She seemed to have more energy and strength and felt better all around. With each treatment, she improved tremendously, and fortunately she did not suffer any of the classic side effects such as hair loss, night sweats, vomiting, swollen legs, nausea, etc. After eleven months, she was released from all further treatments and was declared to be absolutely free of all cancer. She knew it from the way she felt.

ELIMINATING BOWEL GAS

If you should happen to have extreme bowel gas, it would make sense to eliminate from your diet some of the things which contribute to bowel gas. As an example, eliminate beans, peanuts, and too much roughage, which are all known to cause gas. Animal proteins such as ground up meat as found in hamburgers, sausages, hot dogs, and some cold cuts should be eliminated.

If animal foods such as hamburgers, fish, etc are eaten, it would be a good idea to consume a sufficient amount of high fiber foods to help decrease transit time and eliminate these foods from the colon before putrefaction can become a gas producing problem.

Mint tea or an extract of mint may help reduce gas, and wild yam extract may be very helpful. If you have irritable bowel syndrome, you may drink flaxseed tea with a teaspoonful of liquid chlorophyll and this may be very helpful.

PROBIOTIC TREATMENTS FOR GAS

You've probably heard lots of antibiotic, but have you ever heard of probiotic? These are the friendly bacteria that reside in your gastrointestinal tract. Probably the best known probiotic is the lactobacillus acidophilus. If it is to be effective, it must contain at least 200 million organisms per cubic centimeter. Clinicians claim that in order to be effective, it must be taken in large doses, but doses as small as 4 ounces daily have worked if mixed with like amounts of supplemental lactose. (NOTE: Lactose is an enzyme that catalyzes the conversion of lactose into glucose and galactose.)

CANCER TREATMENTS MAY CHANGE IN FUTURE

Inasmuch as this IPT treatment is new to most doctors, you may have to contact the medical association in your state in order to find a doctor who can give this type of treatment. I would certainly recommend this in preference to most other treatments since it works, and it also doesn't take so very long for good results to be known. Of course, if you can't afford it, you may have to try something that does cost less. We know that most insurance companies will not pay for this or for any other treatment which is not of the cut, burn, or poison type. It seems to me that some insurance company will eventually learn that it costs less for many of the alternative treatments than the conventional treatment, which is very ineffective and very costly. They could save money using other systems, but it may take another 20 or 30 years for them to catch on to this.

If you are able to find a doctor who can and does successfully treat you for your cancer, I hope you will write to me and tell me all about it. I care!

THE BEST TREATMENT

Dr. Richard Schulze, the world's greatest doctor, used a very special treatment for all his patients who came to his clinic for treatment. He had every person go on a juice fast for usually 30 days and they could drink all the freshly squeezed orange juice or other juices and drink as much herbal tea with honey as they wanted. In addition, each patient took Intestinal Cleansers #1 and #2, Echinacea Plus and SuperFood. You will read more about these four items in Chapter 3 of this book.

Chapter Three

The Colon

When Dr. Richard Schultze first started his medical practice, he says "God sent me a lovely, but very depressed, woman patient about 50 years old. She was partially depressed because of anxiety of menopause, but mostly because of her daughter.

I had heard from another patient that her daughter had a chronic bowel problem, so I asked her to tell me about it, and she told me this story.

Her daughter always had trouble going to the bathroom since she was an infant, but when puberty arrived, her bowel just about stopped working altogether. For two years she hardly went to the bathroom at all. At 15, after suffering very long bouts of constipation, and almost constant pain in her lower abdomen, she finally developed diverticulitis (an infected, herniated, irritated, inflamed, painful bowel) with colon and rectal bleeding. Since medical doctors know nothing about herbs and their healing ability, not even Aloe Vera, they resorted to going up inside this little girl's rear end a few times and cauterized (burned) the inside of her colon in a last ditch effort to stop the bleeding. Finally after six months of torture, they suggested the removal of her bowel, a colostomy, and said it would save her years of future suffering.

The doctors convinced the family that this was a fairly simple procedure and that many people live a normal comfortable life after having a colostomy. When the daughter woke up after the surgery in the hospital with no bowel, a big red sutured scar from one side of her belly to the other and a hole the size of a silver dollar in her gut with a plastic bag glued on it filled with poop, well she was quite freaked out as you can imagine. The doctors said she would get used to it in no time, but she didn't. After months of depression and not wanting to go to school, her mom decided to throw her a sweet sixteen party to lift her spirits.

They invited all of her friends, including a new boyfriend she met at the mall. Mom even sprung for a new party dress. The night of the party came and everything was going great. Towards the end of the party, her daughter was slow dancing with her new boyfriend, they kissed, it was perfect. Then all of a sudden, he shrieked and pushed her away in terror He was covered with hot, wet stinking fecal sludge and so was she. Her bag had become unglued and fell off, spurting its contents everywhere, covering her, her new party dress, and her new boyfriend.

Needless to say, the party was over and the daughter ran to her room in a hysterical, sobbing, crying fit. Mom cleaned her up and tried to console her, but finally decided to let her sleep it off, thinking that tomorrow would be a new day. When mom went up to her daughter's room in the morning, her daughter had hung herself in her closet, she was dead. So much for what the doctors call a simple surgery."

Dr. Schulze interrupted to make a statement he felt he had to say. He said, "Some people think that I am acting too much like a hard ass when I call the A.M.A. the American Murderer's Association. Well if they would have spent a few weeks in my clinic, seeing all the little children tortured and killed, they'd call them a lot worse."

Then he continued, "As God works, the very next day I got a call from another frantic mom, except this time it wasn't too late. It was Tuesday and the mom told me that her little 11 year old boy was scheduled for a colostomy surgery (colon removal) on Friday. He had been constipated for years and had not gone for months. She begged me to help, but I only had two days in which to work a miracle. I put together a very strong experimental herbal bowel cleanser, because none of the ones my teachers taught me had ever worked for any of my seriously constipated patients. So I got out my old veterinary herbals from the 1800s and looked up what they would use for large animals like horses, picked out a few herbs, mixed them up, and I gave them to this boy and the very next day he had a bowel movement. Mom called me and told me it was over two feet long and up to 2 to 3 inches wide. It was so hard that after numerous attempts at flushing it down the toilet, her husband had to go out to the garage and get a shovel and had to chop it up to get it to flush. This kid is now a grown man, married and with two kids of his own. How much do you think his life would have changed, if not ruined, had he undergone that horrifying, disfiguring surgery?

From this day on, I vowed to never let another child, or ANYONE suffer from constipation or have a mutilating colon surgery. But all I had to work with were outdated and antique herbal formula.

What I used on this little boy was the first crude version of my Intestinal Corrective Formula #1. Until I refined it, some friends referred to it as TNT Herbal Explosive and Depth Charges. I am strongly against animal torture and experimentation, but I needed to refine my formula. This is when I discovered that relatives are often a great inexpensive replacement for laboratory rats. I gave one of my earliest versions of this formula to my brother, who had a long history of constipation... well not anymore. I made a mistake with my calculations and gave him a serious overdose. He not only experienced the laws of jet propulsion, but claims that he has had perfect bowel movements for the last 25 years. I eventually got the formula smoothed out.

HOW MUCH FECAL MATTER CAN A PERSON HOLD?

The average American stores from 6 to 10 pounds of fecal waste in his colon, which is not healthy. As far as the record breaking accumulation of fecal matter, I had one man in Hawaii who got his dosage up to 46 capsules of my Intestinal Corrective Formula #1, (that is a record itself), before his bowels moved. Then that night, sitting on the toilet, HE EVACUATED 56 POUNDS OF FECAL MATTER. I met his wife and she said to me that "she always knew her husband was full of shit," (her words, not mine), but she was right. I had one lady that after a year of my herbal bowel cleansing program lost over 200 pounds. She went from over 410 pounds down to 180.

A CLEAN COLON MAY HELP PREVENT CANCER

Looking under a microscope, anyone can see parasites in animal food. One cubic inch of beef often has over 1,000 parasite larva in it. Fish is the worst, some of their parasites are as big as earthworms. There are even many parasites that live on fruits and vegetables, but if a person has 2 or 3 bowel movements a day, these parasite larva don't hatch, and you're fine. And if you're like me and eat lots of garlic, well no self-respecting parasite is going to take up house in your colon anyway.

But if you don't have regular bowel movements and only go a few times a week, well these parasite larva hatch, hook onto your colon and start feeding on your backed up waste and even feed on your tissue. In my clinic I had every patient do my bowel detoxification program, which is a real parasite flush. After doing it, they would bring in bottles, jugs, and pails full of worms, some of them quarts of little worms, many the size of snakes. One of my patients actually went to the hospital after doing my bowel detoxification program because of colon pain. Later the hospital called me to report that she had evacuated a 35 foot tape worm. WOW!

HOW BAD CAN IT GET? MY CONSTIPATION RECORD BREAKERS

Thirty years ago, when I first heard Dr. Christopher speak about extreme constipation, I thought he was lying. (Note by Author: Dr. John R. Christopher was one of the all-time great medical doctors who lived until 1983. He died from an injury received in a fall, and he was 82 years old then, as I recall. Dr. Schulze learned a great amount of his medical information from Dr. Christopher as well as Dr. Bernard Jensen, who died in 2001 at the age of 92.) I wanted to believe him, but when he started telling me that he had patients that hadn't had bowel movements in a month, well now I thought he was telling me a natural healing fish story.

But in the first year of running my Hollywood clinic, I had a fashion model come to see me, a very beautiful girl, slim, 5'8" and 115 pounds, and she only had ONE BOWEL MOVEMENT A MONTH for the last year and a half. I was shocked. Where did it go? I was ready to call David Copperfield or Sigfried and Roy. This was real magic.

That year I had many patients that only had one bowel movement a month and for a few years in the clinic that was the record until a woman came to see me, a 38 year old attorney that only went every other month. She had ONLY 6 BOWEL MOVEMENTS IN A YEAR! She held the record for a while, but then there was a young woman from Santa Rosa, California. She only had 3 bowel movements during her last pregnancy. That's one bowel movement per trimester and only two others that year. That held the record for some time, but two years ago I got a letter from a lady in Southern California thanking me for my Intestinal Formula #1. In the letter, she stated that before using my herbal formula, she was only having one bowel movement every 6 months. THAT IS ONLY 2 BOWEL MOVEMENTS A YEAR, THE CURRENT RECORD HOLDER!!!!

Sure the above were extreme cases, but most of my patients suffered from some sort of constipation. I had well over a thousand patients that were lucky if they went once a week. People who are constipated live in discomfort, fear, and shame. They usually don't go around talking about it and don't know where to turn. Everyone has failed them, the empty promises of their medical doctors, the wimpy herbal laxatives that couldn't even make you fart, and the natural healers with their bran, give me a break. They pay money, and could fill a bus with the bottles of drugs and herbs that they took. BUT THEY STILL COULDN'T POOP UNTIL THEY MET ME.

WHAT THE HECK IS A NORMAL POOP ANYWAY?

I have literally traveled around the world in search of what a normal bowel movement and bowel habit should be like. Now how many people can say that? I have traveled from the remote jungles of Central America to India, China, almost everywhere to discover what is normal because I knew I wasn't going to find normal in New York, California, and not even in Iowa. I wanted to see primitive people living in rural non-industrialized areas, living simple, natural rural lives under very little stress, getting moderate amounts of exercise and eating simple, natural diets of locally foraged food. These relaxed primitive people all seemed to have one bowel movement within 20 to 30 minutes after each major meal that they ate. They just squat, it rapidly comes out within a minute, and they are done. No library of magazines, no squeezing, straining, grunting, meditation or prayer, it just came out effortlessly. They seem to average between 2 and 4 bowel movements a day, or 14 to 28 bowel movements a week compared to the average American's bowel habit of 1 bowel movement every 3 to 5 days or 2 to 3 bowel movements a week. I FIGURED THIS PUTS THE AVERAGE AMERICAN ABOUT 70,000 BOWEL MOVEMENTS SHORT IN HIS LIFETIME!

NORMAL CONSISTENCY

The consistency of your bowel movements should be soft and unformed like peanut butter or soft serve frozen ice cream. Occasionally they can be a bit chunky depending on what you ate and how well you chewed it, but in any case, they should not be formed and they should be light in color. I remember as a kid my dad only went once a week on Sundays. He would take the entire Sunday paper in the bathroom and he would be in there for hours. When he came out, the room smelled like someone died. I would then take my place at the throne after him and squeeze hard for my once a week bowel movement. Eventually I would blast out some small black balls as hard as granite. My dad would come into the bathroom to wipe me, but my fecal matter was so dry and hard there was nothing on the toilet paper. I remember my dad remarking, "Now that's a good poop, no wiping, like it's wrapped in cellophane" and I would leave for a week thinking I did a good job.

SIGNS OF CONSTIPATION

If you need a library in your bathroom, you know, like a stack of magazines on the hamper, then you are constipated. If you drink coffee, well if you stop, you will also probably stop having bowel movements too.

MY PATIENTS TAUGHT ME THE POWER OF COLON CLEANSING, IN SPITE OF MYSELF

Like any great egomaniac student in herbal college, I wanted to develop very intricate and detailed herbal formula. These herbal formulas would be very difficult to make and could only be made from very exotic and rare herbs found only in the rain forest or in the Himalayas. And of course, these formulas would be extremely effective for treating very specific diseases. I was going to find the herbal cure for cancer.

Thank God my great teachers deeply ingrained in me that before I could embark on any of my disease specific smart bomb herbal fantasies, I must get my patients on a good health program, first things first. First I needed to get them following the basics for a month or two, what I now refer to as my Foundational Programs, the foundations of health. A good clean, and wholesome food program, thorough bowel cleansing and detoxification, immune boosting, exercise and positive emotional work. I knew that there was no replacement for these basics.

By doing so, I unknowingly destroyed my fancy, disease specific, herbal formula dream because approximately 80% of my patients, regardless of what was wrong with them, regardless of how long they had been sick, they got more than relief, THEY GOT WELL from just bowel cleansing! When I added the other foundational programs, over 90% got well with no specific treatment at all. So much for my trips to Tibet.

You heard right, the vast majority of my patients got well and recovered from their disease without any specific treatment. All they did was make some common sense lifestyle changes, including cleansing the bowel, and they were healed. My patients, having the nerve to get well before I was ready, ended all my dreams of discovering herbal cures for the afflictions of mankind and turned me into the common sense herbal country doctor that I am today.

BOWEL CLEANSING CAN BE THE CURE FOR ANY DIGESTIVE DISEASE

Bowel cleansing can be very effective for any disease, but especially diseases of the digestive tract. I had many patients heal their upper gasto-intestinal problems like ulcers, hyperacidity, gastric reflux, hiatal hernia, and indigestion, to colon problems such as chronic constipation, to spastic colons, colitis, and Crohn's disease, and yes, even hemorrhoids. Even liver and gall bladder problems are often relieved because the same herbs that cleanse and detoxify the bowel also stimulate, cleanse and detoxify the liver and gall bladder.

Many people write me and ask about polyps and bowel cancer, which often go hand in hand. Although I am banned from telling you about my specific patients healing their serious bowel diseases, like cancers, here is a story I got from an American Botanical Pharmacy customer in San Diego, California, a few years ago. He was in his 60s, and because of a family history of degenerative bowel disease and colon cancer, his son asked him to go to the doctor and get a sigmoidoscope check, a look into the bowel. This is getting to be a routing check now for older folks to look for bowel cancer and bowel disease.

Well sure enough they saw it, a big cancer they said looked like a big mushroom, growing in his sigmoid colon, and it had metastasized and invaded into the muscle, maybe even farther. He also had around 35 polyps. The doctor wanted to admit him immediately to the hospital for a colon resection. They wanted to gut him and carve out at least 12 inches of his colon, probably more. He was very scared.

His son suggested that his dad do my bowel cleansing program. The father asked the doctor if he could delay the colon surgery for a few months while he did an herbal bowel cleanse. The doctor said he was nuts, the herbs could be dangerous and even if they weren't, they were useless and that a delay of a few days, let alone months, could be suicidal. The cancer would just grow worse, spread, metastasize, and kill him.

The dad told me he was more afraid of the doctors and their surgery. So he decided to do my Bowel Detoxification Program. After 8 weeks of bowel cleansing, using 8 entire jars of Intestianl Corrective Formula #2, 3 bottles of Intestinal Corrective Formula #1, double daily doses of SuperFood, and lots of Echinacea Plus, he went back for another look by the doctor. The doctor was furious, and said that surgery may not save him now because he delayed getting proper professional treatment by playing around with some hocus-pocus herbs. BUT WHEN THE DOCTOR LOOKING INTO THE COLONOSCOPE, HE LITERALLY SHRIEKED, 'OH MY GOD, I DON'T BELIEVE IT.'

Not only were all 35 polyps gone, disappeared, not a trace of even one, but the cancer looked like a dried up skeleton of a cancer. (This is exactly what cancer looks like after your body and especially your white blood cells eat up a tumor.) He said the doctor then touched the cancer skeleton with a tool through the scope and that it just fell off the bowel. THE CANCER JUST FELL OFF.

I had hundreds of patients with bowel polyps that got rid of them. I had many other patients with bowel cancers that disappeared. I had other patients with supposedly unrelated problems like clinical depression, dementia, arthritis, neurological diseases, the list is endless, that all got relief from doing a thorough bowel cleanse.

DR. SCHULZE'S INTESTINAL DETOXIFICATION PROGRAM

INTESTINAL CORRECTIVE FORMULA #1 (Cathartic Formula)

Contains: Curacao and Cape Aloe leaf, Senna Leaves, and Pods. Cascara Sagrada aged bark, Barberry root bark, Ginger rhizome, Garlic Bulb and African Bird Pepper.

Therapeutic Action: This stimulating tonic is cleansing, healing and strengthening to the entire gastro-intestinal system. It stimulates your peristaltic action (the muscular movement of the colon) and over time strengthens the muscles of the large intestine. It halts putrefaction and disinfects, soothes and heals the mucous membrane lining of your entire digestive tract. This herbal tonic improves digestion, relieves gas and cramps, increases the flow of bile which in turn cleans the gall bladder, bile ducts and liver, destroys Candida albicans overgrowth and promotes a healthy intestinal flora. It also destroys and expels intestinal parasites, increases gastro-intestinal circulation and is anti-bacterial, anti-viral and anti-fungal. Continue to use this formula until you are having at least 1 bowel movement for each meal that you eat. Between 2 and 4 bowel movements a day is normal. Considering all the disease and death we have because of retained fecal matter, I wouldn't worry about taking too much of this formula.

Patient Type A: The sluggish bowel type. This formula is for 97% of my patients, the ones who need help getting their bowel working more frequently. You must use this herbal formula every day to keep your bowels very active.

Dosage: Start with only 1 capsule of this formula during or after dinner. This formula works best when taken with food or juice. The next morning you should notice an increase in your bowel action and in the amount of fecal matter that you eliminate. The consistency should also be softer. If you do not notice any difference in your bowel behavior by the next day, or if the difference was not dramatic, then that evening increase your dosage to 2 capsules. You can continue to increase your dosage every evening by one capsule until you notice a dramatic difference in the way your bowel works. There is no limit. Most people only need 2-3 capsules, but a few have needed over 30 capsules. It has taken most of us years to create a sluggish bowel, so let's be patient for a few days and increase by only 1 capsule each day.

Patient Type B: The irritated bowel type. This only applied to a small percentage of my patients. These are the exceptions to the rule, those with bowels that move too often (more than 3 times a day). This includes those with Colitis, Irritable Bowel Syndrome, Crohn's Disease, etc. If your bowels are irritated, hot or working too frequently, skip this formula and go to Intestinal Correctional Formula #2.

INTESTINAL CORRECTIVE FORMULA #2 (Drawing and Detoxifying Formula)

Contains: Flax seed, Apple Fruit Pectin, Pharmaceutical Grade Bentonite Clay, Psyllium seed and husk, Slippery Elm inner bark, Marshmallow root, Fennel seed and Activated Willow charcoal.

Therapeutic Action: This cleansing and soothing formula is to be used in conjunction with Intestinal Formula #1. This formula is a strong purifier and intestinal vacuum. This formula draws old fecal matter off the walls of your colon and out of any bowel pockets. It will remove poisons, toxins, parasites, heavy metals such as mercury and lead and even remove radioactive material such as Strontium 90. This formula will also remove over 3,000 known drug residues and toxic chemicals. Its mucilaginous properties will soften old hardened fecal matter for easy removal and make it an excellent remedy for inflammation in the intestines such as diverticulitis or irritable bowel. Many persons discovered that this formula also removed their colon polyps. This formula is an antidote for food poisoning and other types of poisoning. Therefore, I always have it with me when I travel.

Before beginning Intestinal Corrective Formula #2, your bowels should be moving at least 3 times a day or at least once for each meal you eat. Continue using Intestinal Corrective Formula #1 until this is achieved.

Dosage: Take Intestinal Corrective Formula #2 five times a day. Mix one heaping teaspoon of Intestinal Corrective Formula #2 powder with 8 ounces of juice or distilled water in a jar with a lid. Shake vigorously and drink immediately. Take anytime during the day. Just be sure to allow about 30 minutes before or after meals, juices or taking your tinctures.

Helpful hint: Put a small amount of water in your jar first. Then add the powder and shake. Then add more water. This keeps the powder from sticking to the jar and making it easier to clean.

This formula contains bentonite clay and may be binding. Type A's may need to increase the dosage by one of the Intestinal Corrective Formula #1.

Type B's may need to take one Intestinal Corrective Formula #1 in the evening if you find you are a little constipated.

NOTE: (by author) You may order the Intestinal Corrective Formula #1 and #2 by telephoning 1-800-HERB-DOC. Dr. Schulze is very generous and usually offers you a free gift with your order. I have already received several nice gifts from him, such as his book, "There Are No Incurable Diseases," which normally costs $12.00. He also runs specials wherein you may order package deals at good discounts. Be sure to ask about them when you order, if you don't already know what is being offered. You may be able to buy package deals of two, three, or even four items together. I would suggest that you buy Intestinal Cleanser #1, #2, Echinacea Plus and SuperFood.

If you decide to take the 30 day juice fast and stay home from work to treat your cancer, you may wish to also order the necessary ingredients to have a liver cleanse and a kidney cleanse. These treatments should also help you to improve your health and are highly recommended by Dr. Schulze.

Chapter Four

The Doctor's Greatest Secret

When I wrote the book entitled "How To Obtain A Fair Trail," I included a chapter entitled "The Lawyer's Greatest Secret," which is a big help to anyone trying to handle his own case. It is also a great help to anyone who contemplates going into business since this secret is used either deliberately or unknowingly by each person who successfully launches a business. Now I want to give you the doctor's greatest secret, which may help you not only to get well but to stay well.

I have no idea what percentage of medical doctors know this great secret, but I would guess that only a few know it. Dr. Richard Schulze accidentally discovered it when he was treating his patients. He was preparing to use his great knowledge treating his patients with herbs for cancer and other ailments. He had learned that before he could embark on any of his disease specific smart bomb herbal fantasies, he must first get his patients on a good health program. To his great surprise, about 80% of his patients got well just because they had gone onto the good health program, and after he added his other foundational programs, over 90% GOT WELL with no herbs or drugs, but I want you to read his story in his own words.

"Get Well" by Dr. Richard Schulze

Colon Cancer KILLS more while media blackout succeeds.

What makes hot news isn't necessarily an accurate reflection of what is really going on in the world. This is especially true when it comes to what people are dying from. So while black tie galas are being held all over America to raise money for breast cancer research, while October has been declared national breast cancer awareness month, while the word mammogram is on every woman's lips, while every man is dreading his next prostate exam, while every magazine you pick up has an article on prostate cancer, and every day there is another article on AIDS, and if that isn't enough I just received an invitation to a black tie gala in New York, "Penthouse Pets bare their breasts for Breast Cancer." I am NOT kidding, and while all our attention is on breasts, the prostate and sex, colon cancer KILLS more men and women in America than Breast cancer, Prostate Cancer, and it actually kills 400% more people than AIDS!

Yes, according to the Center for Disease Control (CDC) death from AIDS has declined significantly in the last 5 years, it's down a whopping 70%, but the AIDS media blitz still continues, SEX SELLS. Many reporters have told me that no one wants to hear about poop and that breasts, prostates and sexual diseases are more sexy and sex related and, therefore, more newsworthy. But sexy or not, AIDS kills about 15,000 Americans a year, prostate cancer will kill about 39,000, breast cancer will kill about 40,000 but Colon-Rectal Cancer will kill about 60,000 American's this year, with over 125,000 new cases diagnosed. I know, I've heard all the excuses, it's dirty, it's embarrassing, and I don't want to talk about poop, or my favorite, I'm too busy to be going to the bathroom all the time. Like ostriches with our heads buried in the sand, we don't want to discuss colon disease or health.

Although Colon-Rectal Cancer and Disease is reported in most modernized countries, America's high levels of constipation and our unwillingness to talk about it has helped us win the international contest hands down. We have now awarded ourselves the highest incidence of Colon cancer and disease of any other country in the world. And according to medical statistics, EVERY American will develop some type of colon cancer, tumor, polyp or disease in their lifetime, so it is high time we started talking about what's causing it and how to prevent it.

Let's Check what the top Medical Doctors Say

The Merck Manual is written by the most distinguished and respected group of top medical doctors in the world and published by one of the largest pharmaceutical manufacturers in the world. It is the medical industry's standard text for the diagnosis and treatment of disease. This book tells us that colon degeneration is on the rise.

The incidence of diverticulosis (herniated bowel pockets caused by constipation) has increased dramatically over the last 50 years. It states that in 1950 only 10% of adults over the age of 45 had this disease, in 1955, 15%, in 1972, 30%, and in 1987 almost half. The latest edition states that the incidence increases rapidly over the age of 40 and that every person will have diverticulosis if they live long enough.

Every American eventually has Diverticulosis or many Diverticula. Diverticula, sac like herniations through the muscular wall of the colon that are caused by increased pressure in the bowel from constipation. By old age every American has many. They are filled with trapped fecal sludge, they become infected, the rotting feces erodes the surrounding mucousa and blood vessels and bleeding, rupturing and infection begins.

Up to 50% of Americans have Polyps in their Colon. A Polyp is a tumor that arises from the bowel surface and protrudes into the inside of the colon. Most polyps eventually transform into malignant cancer tumors.

So while the top Medical Doctors are saying that Bowel Disease is more prevalent than ever, and killing more Americans than ever before, why don't I see more Bowel Detoxification Programs in all the new natural healing books being published? It appears that Natural Healers and these modern day hip medical doctor authors have politely swept it under the carpet and consider it dirty or not high tech. It's like they forget that we even have a bowel. They would rather discuss the latest enzyme fad to lose weight or debate how melatonin helps jet lag. The most popular diets today like the Zone (eat the hamburger but throw the grain bread out) and the Atkins (heavy animal protein blood-feast) are almost fiberless regimes that left most of my patients constipated to the gills with severely increased cholesterol levels. There is no shortage of hype on St. Johnswort, Cats Claw, Kava Kava, Colloidal Silver or the latest lose weight amino acid craze, sam-e, but what about the foundation of health, having a clean colon, has it become politically incorrect to discuss the bowel? While these so-called health authors ignore colon cleansing and won't discuss it, millions of Americans are literally rotting from the inside out.

I will never forget my first year in practice. I had already healed myself, and I had spent ten years traveling around the country following, studying and interning with the best natural healers and herbal doctors of the last century. I attended their schools, graduated most of them, received two doctorates, 17 different diplomas in all and went on to teach at most of these same schools. To earn money to eat and pay tuition I worked in most of their clinics and saw patients on the side in massage studios, book stores and the back rooms of health food stores. But now the year was 1975 and I thought I knew everything, I was definitely over-trained, under-experienced, and armed with my teacher's herbal formula, I unleashed myself on the world and set up my first real practice in Hollywood, California. But I am afraid nothing could have prepared me for my patients.

I had a lady come to see me; she had been out of work, literally flat on her back in pain for 2.5 years. She had pain in the lumbar vertebrae, sacrum and sciatic nerve. EVERY DAY, ALL DAY. No work, not even housework, not even going shopping for a few groceries, she was 100% crippled, a total wreck. The medical doctors wanted to fuse her spine, maybe even cut the sciatic nerves to relieve the pain. This is a total dead end. She had many visits to her Chiropractor along with Hatha Ycga, which are two of the best therapies for any spinal problem, and especially lower back problems, but she got little results. The Osteopaths or Orthopedic treatments didn't help either and she was at her wit's end. She even told me that she was contemplating killing herself.

Guess what, she was constipated! I put her on the bowel-cleansing program and in less than a week all her pain was gone, and never returned. She was shocked, in disbelief. And she was really, really mad at all the coctors for overlooking something so simple, constipation. Her blocked, engorged, swollen colon was pressing on all the nerves in her lower back.

So even if a person thinks that his particular problem is unrelated to the colon, he might be wrong. A swollen, constipated, irritated bowel puts pressure on and infects everything around it. The nerves from the spine, run right next to the bowel before they go down the legs. I have had hundreds of patients with chronic back pain, sciatica, leg pain, and it all disappeared after a good bowel cleansing program.

No matter how far removed the problem seems from the colon, no matter how ridiculous it may seem to do a bowel cleansing program instead of brain surgery, cleanse the bowel first and see what happens.

"How could so many seemingly unrelated health problems be caused by constipation? To answer this question let's take a quick peek at the inside of your body."

I remember when my older brother got his first car, it was a 1950 Ford station wagon. Of course it didn't run, what kid's first car did. So it sat in our driveway and we would sit in it dreaming of the day when we would be burning rubber down the highway. Being more mechanically inclined, I did most of the work on it to get it running. I used to be able to open up the hood, sit on a front fender with my feet and legs actually dangling inside the engine compartment and work on the engine, change spark plugs, whatever. Get the picture, big car, big hood, little engine, lots of room. Nowadays, I open up the hood of my

1998 Ford Expedition and I just shut it right back up. Every square inch under the hood is jammed, packed with engine parts, power pumps, wires, hoses, pipes, filters, it is too complex, and even if I understood it, there is NO ROOM to work on it. NO SPACE!

What's my point? I used to think our anatomy was like our brother's 1950 Ford, you know a lung up here, a kidney way down there, a bowel in the middle, with lots of room. Then one day in school I examined my first cadaver and WOW, what an enlightening experience. The human anatomy is not like my brother's 1950 Ford at all, it is like my 1998 Ford, every square inch is packed with something and everything is touching something else. This body of ours must have had some incredible engineer. Everything has its place and THERE IS NO EXTRA ROOM! If one organ swells or gets bigger, then another organ, usually the one next to the swelling one gets squeezed, compressed or crushed. Organs don't work so well when they are crushed and the blood, lymphatic, nerve and general circulation gets interrupted. Every organ needs to get nutrition to get waste out in order to be healthy. Squeezed and compressed organs get sick.

Now the entire colon is so big, that it is connected to, touches, sits next to or is in the vicinity of every major organ in the human body, except the brain. It also touches most of your major blood vessels and nerves. Constipation causes the colon to literally swell, expand and even herniate. Remember that the leading medical books told us that all of us store too much fecal matter and have this happening inside of us. So when an area of the colon gets constipated, and swells, it compresses and crushes the organ next to it. This could be the lungs, the heart, the liver and gall bladder, the pancreas, the kidneys and adrenals, the uterus, the prostate, again, almost every major organ in the body. This is simply why a constipated swollen colon can cause an almost endless amount of seemingly unrelated diseases and problems, and I haven't even discussed toxic build up in the colon that literally infects and poisons the nearby organ.

The majority of my patients in my clinic were female. Many women could never understand the relationship between their painful periods, P.M.S., menstrual irregularity, vaginal infections, infertility, menopausal problems, problems during pregnancy, whatever, and their constipation until I explained that their sigmoid colon wraps around the uterus and that their ovaries are literally attached to the colon. The cure for almost every female problem in my clinic besides my Female Formulae was a good bowel cleansing.

Men, don't try to wriggle out of this one, it's the same for you and your prostate, which is attached to your intestines also, and often the part of your colon that gets constipated most often.

The point is that there is NO EXTRA SPACE in your body. If your bowel swells due to constipation and bowel pockets, another organ gets pinched, if not crushed.

What's the bottom line? A sluggish, constipated, swollen bowel, retaining pounds of old fecal matter can either compress a nearby area causing disease or emit infection and toxins which can affect and infect any area of the body.

This explains why many of my patients healed their heart problems, blood pressure problems, breathing problems, blood sugar problems, hormone imbalance problems, fertility problems, liver problems, cholesterol problems, immune problems, urinary problems, adrenal and lack of energy problems, prostate problems, digestive problems, lower back problems, leg circulation and nerve problems by cleaning out their colons before I ever did any specialized treatment for their problem. This explains why so many of my patients healed their almost infinite list of various diseases by doing my Bowel Detoxification Program.

"My patients healed their brain diseases with colon cleansing proving that you can't have sweet thoughts on a sour stomach."

I had many patients with Alzheimer's Disease and many different types of dementia that turned around and healed themselves after a complete bowel cleanse. And I don't mean people who were just a little foggy and forgetful, I had patients who howled like wolves on the full moon, they were totally gone. I had a patient come to me with clinical depression, one of the worse cases I ever saw. He used to be a brilliant man and now he couldn't even speak or get himself dressed.

His family brought him into my clinic where he sat on the couch in the waiting room with his head sunken and glued into his hands. This poor man was frozen stiff and a tow truck couldn't get him into my examination room, so I just sent him home. But I asked the family to start him on the basics, but all they did was my Bowel Detoxification Program.

Over the next few months this man evacuated some ungodly stuff. The family said it stunk up the entire house, even the next door neighbors complained. But to everyone's surprise this man started coming back and within a few months was back to normal and a month or so later back to work. JUST BY CLEANING OUT HIS COLON!

NEVER, NEVER, NEVER, NEVER, NEVER, NEVER, UNDERESTIMATE THE POWER OF COLON CLEANSING. Everyone wants a quick cleanse or a 24 hour detox. Sure, party for a decade and then try to clean up the whole mess in a few minutes, it's not going to happen. Any cleansing or detoxification program is a TOTAL JOKE unless you do a thorough bowel cleansing for a few weeks FIRST!

When any patients came to see me, my eventual goal was to get them to do some sort of detoxification routine; a cleanse. The purpose of a cleanse is to remove toxins from the fat, muscle, blood and internal organs that have accumulated there over a period of years. This is how you prevent disease, by cleaning out these poisons before they make you sick. When you do a cleanse you use herbs to loosen and break up all of this accumulated waste and poison and it now has to flow out of the elimination channels, especially the colon and kidneys. If these elimination organs are not clean and operating properly you can't get the poison out of your body.

First, you obviously will not get the benefit out of your cleanse, but secondly you will feel awful and might even get very ill. See, all of your cleansing and detoxification removed all the poison from your tissues, and now it is sitting in your colon, but can't get out. Chances are you will reabsorb these poisons and feel worse than you did before you started your cleanse. I had so many patients who, before they came to my clinic, had already tried to do their own self-designed cleanse or detox. They would party on the weekend and then start the carrot juice fast on Monday morning. By noon they would have a blinding headache and by dinner they would breakdown and eat pizza. Anyone who has started any type of detox and felt bad within hours needed to do a colon cleanse. This way all the poisons that you are cleaning out of your body, CAN GET OUT OF YOUR BODY. So the first step, before you start a whole body detox, should be the cleaning out and strengthening of the elimination organs, and the bowel is the best place to begin.

Chapter Five

There Are No Incurable Diseases

Dr. Richard Schulze has written a book entitled "There Are No Incurable Diseases" and I believe that this is really powerful information. Of course, it is difficult to believe that AIDS, Alzheimer's, Cancer, Drug Addiction, Malaria, Poor Circulation, and all of the other diseases can be cured. A copy of his book may be purchased from American Botanical Pharmacy, 4143 Glencoe Avenue, Dept. 7, Marina Del Rey, CA 90292 for $12.00 plus shipping. I urge you to buy several copies for yourself and friends who may be ill or dying. It's worth many times the price you will pay and could save your life.

He has a 30 day intensive cleansing program to clean your body internally for starters. Of course, we all know that in order for any cure to ever take place, we must have a sufficient amount of time for the cure to work. If we have at least 30 days left, then we certainly have a good chance, but if we only have minutes, hours, or only a few days, then our chances are almost non-existent. Dr. Schulze has a great detox program to cleanse your system internally both thoroughly and completely. He also advocates a hot and cold shower treatment as well as the cold sheet treatment.

COLD SHEET TREATMENT

Dr. Schulze states that: "Fever is never dangerous if you hydrate the body and get lots of liquid." We know that when our immune systems discover a disease in our bodies, then the area where they are located becomes very hot to destroy the disease. If we take aspirin to stop the fever, we interfere with our immune system's efforts to destroy the disease, bacteria or virus causing the trouble. As our temperatures rise, for each degree that it rises above 98, the speed at which our white blood cells travel as well as their effectiveness is doubled. For example, if our temperature is 99, then the speed is doubled to 2x. At 100, it is 4x, at 103, it is 32x and 104, it is 64x. If you take aspirin, you suppress your immune system to stop it from destroying the disease or problem. It is like taking a boxer, and after tying his hands behind him, sending him into the ring to fight with an opponent. If you suppress your immune system, your disease will make you much sicker, so remember, when you become ill, fever is your best friend and should be protected.

You will not be able to give yourself the cold sheet treatment. You need two people to help you and Dr. Schulze says you should not use your spouse as one of them, unless she is 1000% supportive. He says things come out while you are in the bathtub that you would not want your spouse to hear.

Dr. Schulze lists 24 things which you will need to do the Cold Sheet Treatment, plus several more items for your bed. One of the items requires that you brew 6 to 8 cups of sage, yarrow or ginger tea, which needs to be guzzled, so it should not be too hot. Another item requires that you begin filling the bathtub with hot water, which will sit for about 10 minutes before you get in. You cut up a t-shirt and make a large bag out of it. Then you fill the bag half way and allow room for the herbs to expand. You fill it with the following herbs: one ounce each of Cayenne powder, Mustard seed powder, and also of Ginger root powder. You then tie the bag with string and insert this tea bag into the water of the tub filled with hot water. The color of the water will change to yellow-orange, but you should squeeze the bag many times to help activate the herbs. The fumes of this may choke you slightly or may even gag you because volatile oils will be coming out of the herbs.

Next, fill your enema bag with cool, distilled water, and then take up to half an hour to do a complete high enema or colonic irrigation. Your objective is to empty the rectum of fecal matter. Next, you should liquefy in a blender 8 ounces of water, 8 ounces of organic apple cider vinegar, and 6 to 10 cloves of garlic. You put the liquid in the rectal syringe, and lubricate the rectum and end of rectal syringe with olive oil. Then you insert the syringe, take a deep breath, and try to get the mixture all in at one time. Warning: This will burn and you will want to evacuate promptly. You may need a few minutes to recover from this.

Next, you will get ready to get into the hot bath. You must prepare for this by covering your genitals, anus, nipples, and all extra sensitive areas or wounds with Vaseline. This is important because if you have your genitals on fire, this could totally ruin your treatment. You want to stay in the tub for 20-30 minutes. You may need encouragement to make it for 30 minutes, but you should do your best to do it. After entering the bathtub, draw more hot water as you want to have it as hot as you can take it. You may scream, holler, and yell, but you should stay in the tub if you can for 30 minutes. You start drinking your 6 or 7 cups of tea as you should drink lots of liquid while in the hot bathtub. There is no reason to worry about dehydration due to your fever as you will be consuming lots of tea.

You should drink the tea rapidly and the next cup of tea should be ready before you finish the first cup. You want to drink all of the tea during the 20-30 minutes you are in the tub.

The Cayenne tincture should be ready in case you feel faint or light headed. Dr. Schulze says "you will not faint if you have a dropper full of Cayenne tincture in your mouth. He says that during the first 5 to 10 minutes, you won't feel anything unusual, but then you will start feeling an uncomfortable burning sensation." You will want to get out of the tub soon after this but you must do everything in your power to stay in for at least another 5 minutes, in spite of the burning sensation.

You will need help to get out of the bathtub and they can begin wrapping you in the cold sheet that has been soaking in the bucket with the ice. This sheet will feel good to you. You should stay wrapped in the sheet for 3 hours, or more. The sheets will draw out poisons which have come to the skin's surface due to the hot bath.

This gives you some idea what it is like to take this type of treatment. If you have a minor illness, you may need one treatment during the 30 days program you are on. If you are terminal, you may want treatments at least once a week.

Chapter Six

Overcoming Impotence Naturally

GENETICS, NATURAL HEALING, AND IMPOTENCY

Dr. Richard Schulze had this to say about impotency, natural healing, etc:

"There is usually only one reason for impotency in men and infertility in women- poor health and a toxic system. I just taught them how to get well and they did the rest. One of the first things you learn in the study of human physiology is that the primary function of the human body is to survive, repair, and then to reproduce. Consequently, your body is always repairing you, always healing you, and striving to be the healthiest that it can. This is its job. Another physiological function is that your level of health is determined by two factors. The reaction of your genetics, which is your inherited strength, and inherited healing power, reacting with your lifestyle and living environment. It is important to understand, whether you are healthy or diseased, that your body is ALWAYS doing the absolute best it possibly can to keep you healthy and alive.

Everyone has some inherited physical strengths and inherited physical weaknesses. On a scale of 1 to 10, a person who inherits a lot of genetic weakness could be considered a 1 or 2, while the person inheriting most of his parents' strengths could be considered a 9 or 10. For those people that inherited almost all strong parts, an 8 to 10, well they can party hearty, live life in the fast lane and burn the candle at both ends. They will probably stay reasonably strong and healthy and probably live a long life. The famous drinking, smoking live to be 100-George Burns is a great example of this. He smoked 3 to 4 packs of cigarettes a day and still won an Olympic gold metal in swimming races. Other people, because of their parents' genetic weaknesses and faulty lifestyle, have inherited more weak parts than strong ones, a 1 to 3 on the scale. Their bodies are constantly getting sick, injured and it is a full time job for them to just keep going and stay alive. A slight breeze can give them a cold and almost fracture a bone. Most of us lie somewhere in between a 4 to 7 on the scale. Usually by age 40 to 45, we begin to observe where some of our weaknesses are and begin to modify our lifestyle to compensate for them.

We can also look to our parents and their health and diseases to see what illnesses may lie ahead of us. We can expect a very similar pattern of health, disease, and longevity as our parents unless we modify how we live. This modification of our environment, if it is a negative health destroying influence, can shorten our life span and decrease our resistance to disease. If we change our environment to a more health promoting influence, we can lengthen our life spans and increase our resistance to disease. This was very obvious to me in my clinic because many of my patients who had developed a serious debilitating disease in the 50s had parents in the "Old Country" that were still healthy and strong in their 80s and 90s. My patients that had strong genetics were meeting too much resistance from living the typical American good life.

A simple experiment to prove this theory is gardening. You can take two genetically identical seeds from the same plant, let's say corn, and then plant them in your garden. Give one seed plenty of sunshine, sufficient pure spring and rain water, and feed the soil with your best compost fertilizer and earthworms. This corn will grow as high as an elephant's eye and feed the whole neighborhood. Take the other genetically identical corn seed and plant it in the shade, under a thick tree, in depleted, rocky, hard soil and give it barely enough polluted water. You will be lucky if it even survives and if it does, you will get one ear about the size of the mini-corn in a Chinese restaurant dish. Both seeds were genetically identical, but the outcome was dramatically different. This is the power that environment and lifestyle have on genetics.

GENETICS is our possible potential, LIFESTYLE determines the results!

WHAT CAUSES ALL DISEASE?

Every human body has a blueprint- a schematic of what perfect health is, and is constantly cleaning and repairing itself to obtain the highest level of health possible. So no matter what you have inherited, your body is always doing its best to repair itself. No matter how strong or weak you are, disease and illness are only present when the body runs into more resistance than it has the capability of dealing with.

This resistance or friction consists of accumulated toxins and waste caused by the body's inability to process, detoxify and remove it as fast as you are consuming it. This can be caused by an improper food program, not getting enough nutrition, and eating too much junk food. It can also be attributed to a lack of exercise, which hinders waste removal, from negative emotional patterns, and from a faulty, unhealthy lifestyle.

Disease begins when your body gets overloaded with waste from an unhealthy lifestyle and it can't flush, detoxify, and repair itself fast enough. Health can be recovered simply by slowing down the attack of life destroying habits until it falls below your inherited strength level and healing ability.

THE CURE FOR ALL DISEASE

When you slow down the attack, below your body's healing ability level, your body will respond by beginning to heal itself. Your disease will go into remission, reverse, and you will begin to get well. Often creating a disease takes focused dedicated work, you have to work hard at making yourself sick. Healing yourself is often just a matter of slowing your self-destroying habits below a certain level, getting out of your body's way and letting it do its primary job, repair and healing. I know this may be a radical thought to some, but what if we decided to begin a few healthy habits. Just imagine what powerful, fast healing you could accomplish if you begin some healthy lifestyle changes and healing programs. This is why in the clinic when my patients would stop killing themselves and started just a few healthy habits and herbal tonics, my God, they would EXPLODE into health almost overnight.

Advanced or aggressive healing is not only getting out of your body's way by STOPPING what made you sick in the first place, but also starting to incorporate healthy habits into your life. In doing so, your body responds very quickly.

Sure, your medical doctor can put 20 dollar names to a million different diseases, but there is only one physiological cause and one simple cure. This explains why, for so many decades in my clinic, my patients were able to heal every disease known with broad spectrum natural healing programs, often before the medical doctor's test results were in. This explains why my Foundational Health Programs like my SuperFood, Bowel Detoxification Program, the Liver and Gallbladder Flush, Kidney and Bladder Flush and 5-Day Cleansing and Detoxification Program created powerful health before I could even diagnose the problem, and no matter what was wrong. This also explains why my Incurables Program, the most powerful program in my arsenal, could reverse diseases that modern medical doctors still say there is absolutely no cure for. What they actually mean is that they have found no medical pill cure, but I sure as heck saw my patients recover from the deadliest of these diseases by simply stopping bad habits and simply getting healthy.

MAYBE, ALL IS WELL?

Often Westerners get flustered and frustrated when they travel thousands of miles to the remotest parts of India and Asia only to hear the guru say "all is well." They wanted to hear complex answers to the mysteries of life and all they got was "all is well," all of the time. Well, I am going to say the same thing when it comes to health and disease. There is no big mystery to it, no mystery at all. Simply your body is just constantly responding with its maximum healing ability. Health or disease is just a matter of the amount of resistance or friction your body runs into as it is trying to repair you and maintain a state of wellness.

So it is not a matter of good health or bad disease. It is just what is, what's so, and what you choose to do about it. Therefore "all is well."

IS IT REALLY A DISEASE, OR A BLESSING FROM GOD?

Often what medical doctors call a disease is actually the beautiful way that your body is taking care of you. We have to stop this idea that we need to kill disease- POISON, ATTACK, BURN, CUT. Often the medical approach is that your medical doctor is trying to kill something inside of you and you have to try to live through this war. Are we at war with ourselves, our own bodies? How about just understanding it, nurturing it and feeding it?

If a patient said the doctor diagnosed osteoporosis, I said "wonderful" and my patient was horrified. I know that the body is creating this life saving situation, not a disease. Osteoporosis is wonderful and I will tell you why.

One of the millions of jobs that your body performs is the monitoring and regulation of blood nutrients. Your body constantly monitors your blood calcium level and when it detects that your blood calcium level is too high, it stores your excess calcium in your bones. On the other hand, if your body detects that your blood calcium level is too low, it takes calcium out of your bones. IF OUT RUN OUT OF CALCIUM, YOU DIE; it's that simple. Your heart stops beating and your lungs stop expanding and contracting, you're dead!

Knowing this, if your blood calcium level dips too low, due to dietary insufficiency, bad assimilation, but most likely because you consume too much protein and sodium, your body will begin digesting and dissolving your bones to get the calcium needed. Your body knows that you will be dead without calcium. Your body knows that you can survive with a weakened and fractured skeletal system. You can even survive with hardly any skeletal system, but you can not survive without a heart or lungs. In the first sentence of this chapter, I told you that the first and foremost job of the human body is to SURVIVE- to keep you alive. If the choice is crippled or dead, you body will always chose crippled. It's that simple.

The same is true for all other diseases, regardless of what it may look and feel like. We have to get away from this medical nightmare LIE that your body is going berserk and is going against you or trying to kill you. I can assure you that just the opposite is true. Your body is doing everything it possibly can to keep you alive. Infertility and impotency are no different!

POTENCY AND FERTILITY- SURVIVAL OF THE FITTEST

Whether you believe it or not, it exists. Whether you want to believe it to be God's Divine plan, nature's perfection, or just the unfair treatment of the weak, it doesn't matter. Because every day, every second on this planet, natural selection is taking place. The fundamental process of survival of the fittest is the reality whether you like it or not. From every cell in your body, to the corn fields of Iowa, to the jungles of Africa, the healthy and strong are winning, and the weak are losing and dying.

Simply put, this process is the weeding out of the weak and diseased and the proliferation of the strong. Terminating the life of the weak and diseased and/or ending their ability to reproduce, and promoting the life, future and reproductive ability of the strong, naturally.

The laws of nature are very simple, yet firm. Nature doesn't want to create sickly, weak children any more than it wants weak strains of corn to prosper. This natural selection is nature's way of guaranteeing and promoting stronger and healthier future generations. It wants the strong to survive and the weak not to be born, and if by chance the weak are born, they need to be recycled early.

I know. I know. I know. God and nature can be very politically incorrect. We currently live in a very civilized era where we have to feel guilty and apologize for being healthy, strong and happy. Where the weak, diseased, and the crippled, I mean handicapped, I mean physically challenged, get the preferred parking spaces, bigger bathrooms, and free drugs, and the bums, hobos, and drug addicts, I mean the unfortunate homeless people, roam the best streets in America where we treat them like religious prophets, giving them free food and money because we feel guilty.

So why is it that we are doing our best to honor the unwell, it seems that God and nature are still being so cruel and have turned their backs on the unfortunate? The fact is that God and nature have always promoted that "you reap what you sow" (so stop blaming and quit whining) and that "help comes to those that help themselves," (in other words, take responsibility.) Because in nature, if you snooze, you lose, you can't reproduce and you die.

One of the simplest ways to observe this is with plants. Weak plants get blown over by the wind, get beaten down by the rain, and get eaten up by the bugs. They grow little seed that is genetically weak and within a few seasons, gone forever. On the contrary, strong plants thrive, survive, adapt, produce seed and get even stronger next year. Garlic, one of our most powerful herbs on the planet, is thought to have been one of the weakest at one time. Many scientists believe that the reason it is so potently packed with anti-bacterial, anti-viral, anti-fungal, and numerous other powerful protecting chemicals was because it was so attacked in the past. It learned how to adapt, grew stronger, and thrived while other plants withered and died.

It is the same in the animal kingdom too. Weak, diseased animals produce weaker, more diseased offspring. Eventually these very weak animals, even if they don't get eaten, lose their ability to reproduce. It is the same for the human race.

IMPOTENCY AND FERTILITY- IS IT JUST BAD LUCK OR IS IT BAD LIVING?

Men and women, not unlike plants and animals, as they live in an unhealthy way, get sick and produce weaker, sickly children. When these children grow up, they often continue to live unhealthy lives, which promotes further weakness and disease. Eventually these children give birth to sick or deformed children, or stillborn children, or they abort fetuses and miscarry, or even become sterile, losing their ability to reproduce.

As we have learned, the primary functions of the human body are to repair, survive and reproduce. If your health level falls below a certain minimal point, you lose these basic functions. Earlier while writing about Osteoporosis, I explained that your body often is forced to make choices for you. Well, when you are unhealthy, especially a woman, your body will always choose to protect and save you so sterility/infertility is a protective measure that your body takes, knowing that in your unhealthy state, you may not be able to survive a pregnancy.

Infertility and impotency in women and men is simply a sign of poor health. If you correct the underlying causes of poor health, you will become fertile.

MEDICAL DOCTORS: ARE THEY MIRACLE WORKERS OR THE ANTI-CHRIST?

The instance of impotency and infertility has reached epidemic proportions in America. Millions of men and women are sterile, and, as usual, medical doctors have stepped up to the plate and turned unhealthy living and reproductive ignorance into a multi-billion dollar industry.

Are medical doctors teaching sterile patients how to take responsibility for their health and live healthy lives to become fertile again? Of course not. Armed with fertility drugs, tube drills and laser beams for just ten or twenty thousand dollars, medical doctors will try to force your body to do something that God and nature have denied.

To clarify this issue, just because I am using the terms Anti-Christ, God and nature in the above statement, THIS IS NOT A RELIGIOUS OR MORAL DEBATE. On the contrary, it is simply a scientific one. The bottom line is that your body is protecting you and does not want you to be able to have children and there are very good and very natural reasons for this.

FOR MEN, it is simple. When you are weak, toxic and sick your sperm count goes down. Today, due to modern living, American males have half the sperm count they had 70 years ago. Also when you are unhealthy, your hormone level goes down, your circulation gets clogged, and you lose your ability to get an erect penis. Nature's response to sickness and disease is the loss of reproductive ability, because nature resists and sometimes refuses to allow the procreation of sickness and disease. I know, some of you men are thinking that you are reasonably healthy. Well, think again. Nowadays what most people think is good health I consider a state of managed disease. Losing your ability to procreate, your potency, is a grave sign of bad health.

FOR WOMEN it is twofold. The above that applies to men also applies to you. When you are weak, toxic and sick, your hormone levels become imbalanced. You may stop ovulating, which basically means no release of eggs for fertilization. Even if you ovulate, your uterus may be toxic and infected and may not be able to hold or feed the fetus.

And when you are weak, sick, diseased, unhealthy, obese, anorexic, stressed out, crazy, whatever, a woman's body has a perfect natural safety/survival mechanism that protects you. Your body knows that you are ill, and that any more physical or emotional stress (like carrying a child for nine months) could kill you. One of the most basic functions of the human body is survival, so temporary sterilization is your body's way of protecting you from killing yourself. If a woman does get pregnant, and at the same time gets sicker, often the woman spontaneously aborts the fetus. This again is not a curse but a blessing. Your body knew that your life would be in danger if you went to full term, so it aborts the unborn child to save you. It may also be that your lack of health caused defects in the fetus, and again this is nature's way of weeding out the sick and weak. Would you rather have a deformed, sick, and dying child? Would you rather be dead?

IF GOD AND NATURE ARE SAYING NO, THEN YOU HAVE TO SAY YES.

If you can't have children, then it is time to get to work. In the clinic, I had thousands of couples that were told by every type of obstetrician, gynecologist, and reproductive specialist that they could never have any babies without powerful drugs, surgery, and expensive laboratory procedures. How dare they! How dare these godless butchers claim to foresee the future.

In my clinic, what I experienced is that EVERY couple that wanted children- EVERY ONE OF THEM HAD BABIES. That's right, every couple, no matter what scientific horror stories they were told by their medical doctors, no matter how many miscarriages, no matter how many abortions, no matter how much scar tissue, no matter how long it had been since the last menstrual cycle, no matter how bad their hormones were imbalanced, were able to have children if they were willing to get healthy. I learned never to underestimate the power of natural healing and getting healthy, when it comes to everything from sperm counts and impotency to ovulation and infertility.

Always remember, God and nature both want you to have children. There is nothing more important, because without the ability to procreate, there would be no life at all. All you need to do is get healthy.

DISEASES OF THE MALE REPRODUCTIVE SYSTEM
(And the natural and herbal cures)

ERECTILE DYSFUNCTION

Erectile dysfunction is the inability to attain or to sustain an erection for sexual intercourse. Twenty million Americans are affected. Ten percent of American males can't ever get an erection. Viagra sales have topped 1 billion dollars in spite of the drug's dangerous side effects and associated deaths with it.

The major cause for a man's inability to get an erection are BAD CIRCULATION, HORMONE IMBALANCE, PRESCRIPTION AND STREET DRUG USE, STROKES AND NEUROLOGICAL DISORDERS.

BAD CIRCULATION

As far as bad circulation, this is almost an American epidemic. Just about every one of my patients needed help with circulation, especially as they got older. The #1 herbal tonic when it comes to circulation is CAYENNE.

Cayenne enhances and stimulates the circulation like no other herb. After all, it is the only herb that after ingestion, turns your face red. THAT'S BLOOD. I put my patients with erectile dysfunction on both cayenne tincture and cayenne powder. Start out slowly and increase your dosage as you can tolerate it. Within a month, my average patient would notice an improvement in his ability to get and maintain an erection.

Often, my patients used my formulae for things other than what I designed them for. One such application was the use of my Deep Tissue Oil on the penis for erectile dysfunction. My patients reported that a few drops of Deep Tissue Oil rubbed into the hands first and then rubbed into the penis helped them obtain an erection. This would only make good sense because one of the things that formula does is increase blood circulation to the area it is used on. Since I have put this in print over the years, I have received even more letters attesting to the success of this application. You could think of this as an external Viagra. Many men suggested that it worked better if the wife rubs it on. Again, start with a few drops.

WARNING:

Some of my patients were sold desperate insane ideas by their medical doctors in a last ditch effort to get an erection. Penile injection therapy was one of them. This is where you inject drugs with a needle RIGHT INTO YOUR PENIS. I know, for most men just the thought of this is enough to make you lose your erection. I saw the downside of penile injection therapy in my clinic with the bruised and bleeding penises, infections and persistent irritation.

Another nightmare is the penis implants. This is where an incision is made in the penis and an inflatable balloon type device is surgically implanted. A pump is also surgically implanted under your skin nearby. When you desire an erection, you pump up the device inside your penis. I have never seen these work well and also seen the horrors of the scarring, infection, trauma and drama that they can cause.

Maybe it would be easier to just get healthy?

HORMONE IMBALANCE

Just like women, men get hormonal imbalances too. Although the hormones don't fluctuate monthly like womens' menstrual cycles, they do fluctuate. I developed my MALE FORMULA in the clinic in response to this male hormonal fluctuation and drop in hormones, especially testosterone levels. This tonic stimulates male energy, sexual energy, sexual desire and sexual performance. If erectile dysfunction is caused by a hormonal imbalance or low levels of hormones, this tonic will dramatically help.

Many men with male climacteric or male menopause, the period later in life when a man has a lessened sexual urge, were brought back to life by using the MALE FORMULA. Just when many men came to my clinic and thought it was all over, I got them healthy and on my MALE FORMULA. This rejuvenated their sexual desire and sexual ability.

I blend the most powerful varieties of Ginseng for the base of the male formula. These ginsengs are famous the world over as a men's sexual tonic and their description follows. So many men in my clinic requested concentrated ginseng blend to use as an occasional turbo charger that I created my Super Ginseng Blend.

PRESCRIPTION AND STREET DRUG USE

Often erectile dysfunction is caused by drug use. Many men in my clinic, after coronary bypass surgery or other surgeries, could not get an erection. Often I would track this down to the prescription drugs. Many heart drugs reduce and even eliminate a man's ability to get an erection, especially drugs for circulation and blood pressure. Often when my male patients complained to their medical doctor about their inability to get an erection, they were prescribed anti-depressants.

None of these anti-depressants helped my patients to get an erection, it just made them not care any more. By getting my male patients healthy, off of their many prescription drugs and on the Cayenne Tincture, Cayenne Powder, Male Formula and Super Ginseng Blend, I was able to help them get their erections and sexual energy back.

Most street drugs are no different. They may seem exciting and sexy to the in-crowd, and touted as the happening thing, but most cause temporary erectile dysfunction. This is definitely true of alcohol, cocaine, and heroin. Even habitual marijuana smoking causes erectile dysfunction.

ANATOMY AND PHYSIOLOGY OF THE MALE REPRODUCTIVE SYSTEM

The male reproductive organs produce hormones (testosterone) and spermatozoa which are the male reproductive cells. These organs are also used for sexual intercourse. There are internal and external reproductive organs. The internal organs include the testes (testicles), ductus deferens, seminal vesicles, ejaculatory ducts, and the prostate gland. The external organs include the penis and the scrotum. The two testicles are the male gonads. They are located inside the scrotum, which is a pouch found in most mammals made up of skin and muscle. They produce the spermatozoa, (spermatozoon is the singular), which are the mature male sex cells, and when they combine with the ova in a woman, they produce a fetus. The testicles also produce the male hormone testosterone. The scrotum contains the two testicles and is attached just behind the penis. The two testes (testi is the singular) are approximately 4-5 centimeters (1 ½ to 2 inches) in length and shaped somewhat like a flat egg. Rolled up within each testi are approximately 1000 seminiferous tubules, each of which is almost 1 meter (about 3 feet) in length when stretched out. These tubules begin to produce spermatozoa at puberty. The interstitial tissue that fills the space between the seminiferous tubules contains interstitial cells that secrete the male hormone testosterone. The tubules eventually straighten out in the scrotum, and these straight tubes then carry the spermatozoa to the epididymis. The epididymis is a twisted mass of long ducts, still within the scrotum. Each epididymis is as long a 6 meters (18 feet) when stretched out. The spermatozoa from the testes are stored in the epididymis for 10-20 days.

The average length of the external penis at rest is about 8 centimeters (3 inches). It consists of a cylinder-shaped shaft with a bulb on the end called the glans which contains the urethral orifice (the end of the urethra). The glans is covered with a movable hood called the foreskin. Circumcision is the religious practice of surgically cutting off this end of the penis. NOTE: This is only done in America and in the Jewish community. This is not done in the vast majority of the world. It is usually done in hospitals, where the baby shortly after birth is strapped onto a restraining board and then the end of the penis is incised.

The urethra from the bladder passes through the entire length of the penis and opens to the outside of the body at the end of the glans. Therefore the penis is used both as the final organ for the emptying of urine and also for the expelling of sperm. The shaft of the penis is formed by the corpus cavernosum in the back of a spongy structure called the corpus spongiosum toward the end. These structures are mesh-like and contain lots of empty spaces. When blood from the branches from the central artery of the penis fills these spaces (venous cavities), the penis swells. This is how an ejaculation occurs.

Ejaculation is the ejection of seminal fluid out of the penis. When the penis is stimulated, especially the glans on the end, the copora cavernosa becomes filled with blood and the penis becomes erect. After a period of stimulation, ejaculation begins. In the first stages of ejaculation, the semen and secretions from the prostate enter the urethra. In the second stage, rhythmical smooth muscle contractions, where the prostate and seminal muscles are, force more semen to be discharged and expelled.

DISEASES OF THE FEMALE REPRODUCTIVE SYSTEM
(And the natural and herbal cures)

Over 90% of the patients that visited my clinic were female. There isn't a female imbalance, problem, illness, or disease that I haven't dealt with, and probably a thousand times. The following natural healing programs and herbal formulae are powerfully effective and served my patients and me perfectly for many, many years.

PUBERTY AND SEXUAL MATURITY

In the clinic I had children patients that started, experienced, and completed puberty without a significant bump; on the other hand, their parents barely survived. I don't know why medicine and society make such a big deal about it. Nothing could be more natural than puberty.

It reminds me of all the warnings I received from supposed do-gooders, warning me about the terrible twos that I was about to experience with my son, and when he turned two, it was a great year, as has every year since. Puberty is a great time, and I still remember it well. Let me give you parents a few suggestions that can help you and your children.

#1. Don't make a big deal about it. We are born, we experience all sorts of wonderful things, and then we die. Nothing scares a kid more than a serious or concerned look on their parents' faces. Parents almost always give too much information to kids asking a simple question. When my seven year old son asks how babies are made, I usually say that your mom and I kiss, hug, make love, and then a while later, she has a baby. He usually says O.K., can we play ball now. Answer questions simply and wait to see if you have given enough information before you continue. Always answer your kid's questions honestly to create that bond of honesty. And if you don't know the answer, say you don't know and research the answer together. Often with kids, less is more.

The only difference in puberty is to make sure that you let them know about any big changes ahead of time so nothing is a big surprise. If possible, I believe mom should talk to the girls and dad should talk to the boys so it comes from a place of knowing and experience. Let them know that what they will be experiencing is very normal, happens to everybody, and is a blessing.

You must also understand that puberty is the transition from childhood to becoming an adult, at least physically. Parents should be aware of this and instill the basics of good behavior and good living into a child before puberty so there are solid fundamentals when puberty arrives. When a child reaches puberty and has a hormone surge, not unlike an adult, they will become more intense, intent, powerful, sensitive and definitely more independent. They are physically their own man or woman now, and you are still their parent, but you are also sexual competition. Have fun with it and keep a loose rein on them now. They will make mistakes, party too hardy, and screw up. Didn't you?

In America today, it is very sad that this is the time when far too many kids run away from home, or are thrown out of them. So many, that homeless 15 to 18 year old kids are now an epidemic. These kids are now referred to as "throwaways" not running anymore, because their parents don't want them back. I see them all over the streets in California and often talk to them. They are great kids, usually the trend-setters. I remember in the 60s I was condemned, beat on, and even arrested for my fashion and hair statements, (actually I still am), only to see these statements become adult fashion a few years later.

Look, I don't necessarily think that there is anything wrong with being pushed out of the nest early. I was at 16. In fact, we may baby our children way too long. But children at this age should know that they are loved and they have a place to come back to, not dumped in the streets with their walking papers.

Of all the physical problems I saw with girls and boys entering puberty, it was always caused by either poor nutrition, constipation, and/or unhealthy toxic junk food program. This is why a good food program and a healthy colon should be fundamentals with your children long before they reach puberty.

A SuperFood smoothie in the morning and a dose of Intestinal Formula #1 after dinner for 30 days can make a gigantic difference with a teenager's attitude, and help keep these kids at home. Give it a try.

P.M.S., ABNORMAL UTERINE BLEEDING AND MENSTRUAL DISORDERS

Medical doctors love to dissect, separate, rename, and generally make things much more complex and complicated than they really are. My entire adult life as a doctor has been trying to put all the pieces back together and simplify things for my patients. So while the medical doctors are pulling apart the thousands of different female menstrual disorders, I would like to bring them back together all under one roof and put them either under P.M.S. or Abnormal Menstruation and Menstrual Bleeding.

P.M.S., IT'S VERY REAL

I remember for many years helping my female patients deal with premenstrual syndrome, long before most male medical doctors would even admit that such a disorder existed. In the early years of my clinic, I had hundreds of women patients who were told by their M.D. that there was nothing wrong with them and that it was all in their heads. Subsequently, many were referred to psychiatrists and put on powerful and debilitating psychiatric drugs, turning them into zombies. Even though PMS has been given some attention, at least a few paragraphs, in medical literature for over 50 years, it wasn't until about a decade ago that most medical doctors really started admitting that this disorder existed. Thankfully today, it has gotten tremendous press so that both women and men are aware that it is as real as menstruation for most women.

Medical statistics, based on reported complaints, state that 40% of menstruating women have premenstrual syndrome. Obviously the medical idiots who compiled this number don't have clinics, don't date, or get out very much. Every female patient I ever had, had some type of noticeable change happen to them prior to this period. Granted a few of the healthy ones noticed little or nothing, but the vast majority of my female patients, over 80% had debilitating physiological and emotional trauma at least on and off. My point is that the average American woman, especially between the ages of 25 to 40, has to be aware that just prior to her period, she is physically and emotionally different, if not ill.

WHAT CAUSES P.M.S.?

What causes Premenstrual Syndrome is actually very simple to understand. Prior to menstruation (your period), both of your major hormones, Estrogen and Progesterone, decline. Take a look at a chart that graphs the hormone levels in a typical 28-day menstrual cycle.

NOTE: At this point, it is important that we agree on our counting period. Day 1 is the first day of your menstruation, and day 28 is the last day of your menstrual cycle, and your period would start on the following day, which would be day 1 again. In a 28-day menstrual cycle, your period would be days 1,2,3,4 etc at the beginning and you would ovulate on about day 14.

Your Estrogen and Progesterone levels stay pretty level until just before ovulation. Around day 11, Estrogen levels go up quite dramatically peaking within a day or two and then start to decline. Progesterone levels begin to rise slightly later around day 13 just before ovulation, and peak later in the cycle around day 20. But both Estrogen and Progesterone levels begin to decline around day 20 to 22 and both fall off quite sharply days 24 through 28.

This normal, but quite dramatic reduction in hormones, just prior to the period, is enough to cause premenstrual symptoms. This shouldn't be considered a disease, and for some women, awareness of it and some lifestyle modifications can balance you right out. See my Non-Medicated Awareness treatment in the next section of this chapter. But with most women, because of the typical American junk food program, constipation, general toxic accumulation, lack of exercise, high stress levels, cell phones, etc this normally rapid decline in hormones is more like a dive bomber heading at a battleship, or Niagara Falls. Get the picture?

SYMPTOMS OF P.M.S.

Physically, generally anywhere from 10 to 4 days before the onset of the period, a woman will start to notice the symptoms. They can last for only a few hours, a few days is more usual, and all 10 days is not uncommon. Regardless of the duration, they magically disappear for almost all women immediately on the onset of menstruation. This actually led many medical doctors to believe in a women's head, not only because of the symptom's transitory nature, but also how such debilitating symptoms could literally disappear instantly, in the doctor's waiting room.

Fluid retention is the most typical symptom and is thought to aggravate and even cause many of the other related and almost endless physical symptoms such as edema, weight gain, reduced urination, breast fullness tenderness and pain, headache, vertigo, fainting, easy bruising, cardiac palpitations (heartbeat skips), constipation, nausea, vomiting, changes in appetite, pelvic pressure, backache, acne, and other skin blemishes.

Emotional symptoms, even though I list them second, for the vast majority of my patients, were much worse and more debilitating than the physical ones. After all, everyone has a headache or vomits, but calling your husband or boss a #%!*?# can take a lot longer to recover from. Medical books list the emotional symptoms as irritability, nervousness, agitation, insomnia, difficulty in concentrating, lethargy, depression and fatigue.

I am sorry but this is ridiculous and typical medical bull. This list of emotional symptoms doesn't come close to the emotional nightmares that I watched erupt in my clinic on a weekly basis. It is grossly understated. My list would be extreme sensitivity and irritability to the point of breakdown, crying for no apparent reason, extreme insecurity, and loss of self-worth and self-esteem, total indecisiveness, intense outburst of anger, loss of self-control, and what I referred to in my clinic as existential nausea (feeling sick about your existence).

I had many other patients over the years who physically attacked people, lost their jobs, husbands, children, homes, destroyed their careers, were arrested for assault and spousal battery, even battery on a police officer. That sure beats what the medical doctors describe as a headache.

Women are very tough creatures and even though they may keep a smile on their faces, and grin and bear it better than most men, never forget that during P.M.S. there is a dragon just under the surface ready to spring out for no reason at all.

THE NATURAL SOLUTION TO P.M.S.: NON-MEDICATED AWARENESS TREATMENT

This was a protocol that I developed for all my female patients who suffered from P.M.S. It is to be used hand in hand with their herbal medication below, and over the years I saw this program literally save women's lives and their sanity.

If you know that you suffer from P.M.S. every month, then let's plan on it instead of acting like it's a big surprise every month. So first get a calendar. You are going to have to do this for the herbal medication anyway, so let's get it now. Mark the first day of your period, that is day 1. Whatever your cycle is- 28,30,32- days, it doesn't matter. Just count ahead that many days, say 28, and then count back 10 days, and mark the last 10 days of your menstrual cycle in red, that would be days 18 through 28.

The first step in healing yourself of anything is the awareness that you have it, so these are the days that you potentially have P.M.S. problems. The next step in healing yourself is not setting yourself up for failure, so on these days, no clothes shopping. Even though your edema is barely noticeable to a man nor measurable by a doctor, every mirror you look into becomes a fat mirror, and you will feel like a beached whale trying to fit into a spandex outfit two sizes too small. Don't torture yourself. Also be aware that you are acutely sensitive during this 10 days. When people are just talking at a normal volume, you feel as if they are yelling at you. They are not, so be aware that you are overly sensitive, and therefore you may overreact. Learn to resist the part of you that wants to make anything a BIG DEAL.

You may also be indecisive. A lack of hormones or a hormone crash emotionally can remove your spine also. If your husband says hey, let's go out to eat, where would you like to eat? You won't know. If he says when, you won't know either; if you ever get there and he asks where would you like to sit, you won't have the faintest idea. Knowing your potential indecisiveness, tell your partner at the onset that you would like him to make ALL of the decisions tonight, ALL OF THEM. This will make him feel manly, and take the heat off of you having to be responsible for anything. Even try leaving your purse at home and just walking out the door with the clothes on your back. This is the time to let your man be a man and you be a woman and get taken care of.

Also, during this 10 days, postpone any big meetings you may have with your partner, husband or boss (if possible), until after your menstruation begins. A great way to set yourself up for failure is to discuss the household budget, decorating, or next year's home remodeling, or politics, or the meaning of life. This is not the time for this. You will negotiate badly, and even if you win, you'll lose.

JOKE: What's the difference between a woman with P.M.S. and a religious zealot extremist terrorist... You can negotiate with the terrorist.

This is the time of month to love and accept yourself. Quietly celebrate being a woman. Celebrate being yin, calm, meditative. Love and accept yourself.

Soothing is a great word and mantra during these 10 days. Hot baths, candles, essential oils, soothing music, stretching and breathing classes, long walks, easy chairs, sweat clothes and blankets. Can you get the picture? Sure, I'm always aware that you still have to work and run your life, but plan some extra time for yourself and don't get into anything heavy.

I cannot tell you how many women that this program saved in my clinic. It stopped the fighting and screaming, and I didn't have to bail them out of jail anymore.

HERBAL MEDICATION FOR P.M.S.

This program is to be done in addition to the above Non-Medicated Awareness Treatment. I developed my P.M.S. Tonic in the clinic specifically for my female patients with PMS. Due to big government, it is now called the Female Balance Formula.

This formula is very similar to the female formula described next under Menstrual Disorders and Menopause. Its primary design is to regulate and balance your hormone levels. The Female Balance Formula for PMS has the addition of Diuretic, Nervine and Antispasmodic Botanicals. These additional herbs are added to relieve the symptoms of PMS, to reduce water retention, edema, and sedate, quiet and calm the nervous system.

ABNORMAL MENSTRUAL PAIN AND BLEEDING

In case your medical doctor has labeled you with an abnormal menstrual bleeding name, here are a few of the main ones that you can figure out what the doctor was talking about.

- Dysmenorrhea: excessive pain and cramping during menstruation
- Amenorrhea: the absence of menstruation
- Abnormal Uterine Bleeding: sometimes referred to as Menorrhagia, the excessive duration of bleeding
- Hypermenorrhea: excessive amount of bleeding
- Polymenorrhea: too frequent of menstruation
- Metrorrhagia: between or inter-menstrual bleeding

In the clinic I discovered that there are only 3 reasons for Abnormal Menstrual Bleeding: Hormonal Imbalance, Constipation/Toxicity and Pelvic Inflammatory Disease.

HORMONAL IMBALANCE

Hormonal Imbalance is a major culprit in menstrual illness. When the hormones are imbalanced, as a woman you are imbalanced because the hormones regulate so many metabolic functions. The cause can be the hypothalamus or pituitary in the brain, the ovaries themselves, the uterus and even other endocrine organs like the thyroid, the pancreas or the adrenals. Consequently the medical approach of trying to pinpoint the culprit is as ridiculous as trying to find a needle in a haystack.

I had patients that spent years with medical doctors getting poked, prodded, stuck, blood tests, biopsies and tissue samples, not to mention spending tens of thousands of dollars, only to have the medical doctor throw up his hands and say I don't know.

The natural approach is the only sane approach. Like I discussed in Politically Incorrect, let's support your body, STOP your bad habits, start new healthy ones and use supportive herbal tonics to let your body do what it was designed to do, heal and repair you. For balancing the hormones, I used the Female Formula. Its ability to balance the hormones is nothing short of magical and a true blessing.

CONSTIPATION AND TOXICITY

Constipation and toxicity are major causes of abnormal menstrual bleeding for many reasons. First and foremost it's just a matter of physics. The uterus that is shedding its endometrial lining, which is your period, lies snugly between the colon, rectum and bladder. If you are constipated, which enlarges and herniates your colon and rectum, what do you think happens to your uterus? You guessed it, it gets smashed, squashed and crushed. Now just imagine what will happen when it's time for your period and your uterus is swelling. It is going to hurt. Billions of dollars worth of over the counter drugs are sold to relieve the pain of menstrual cramping. I found in the clinic that my Intestinal Formula #1 and my Bowel Detoxification Program relieved over 80% of my female patients' menstrual cramps, permanently.

There is also the case of toxicity. Again the uterus lies snugly between your colon, rectum and bladder, a tight fit sharing only thin tissue separating them. The same blood vessels interact between these organs. Also, the colon, rectum and bladder are the last holding and storing tanks for the elimination of the 2 major elimination channels in the body, over 95% of the human waste. Also being the last stage of waste, this is where the most poisonous, toxic and infected waste is. It is well known that putrid, toxic and infected material from your colon can seep and leak through sacular herniations called diverticuli.

The bladder can also be a major culprit because often women have bladder infections which are not just restricted to their bladders. Infection spreads in your body from one organ to another. Since bladder infections are extremely common in women, especially sexually active women, I also always had my female patients suffering from menstrual illness do my 5-Day Cleansing and Detoxification Program using the Kidney/Bladder Flush Drink and the Kidney/Bladder Formula and the Kidney/Bladder Tea, for an entire week. This clears up the most stubborn bladder infections and even ones you didn't know you had and eliminates urine aggravation.

The bottom line (pun intended) is that retained diseased waste in the colon, rectum and bladder surrounds and infects the uterus, causing sickness, inflammation, swelling and pain and also Pelvic Inflammatory Disease.

PELVIC INFLAMMATORY DISEASE

Pelvic Inflammatory Disease, referred to as PID, is also a major cause of chronic pelvic pain, ectopic pregnancies and infertility. Over 1 million women are diagnosed with PID every year in America, and it is estimated that millions more have it, at least 1 out of every 6 women.

It can be an infection of the cervix, uterus, the endometrium or uterine lining, the fallopian tubes, the ovaries, or a combination or all of these organs. Vaginal infections alone are generally not considered PID but can easily turn into PID in a few hours. Some old fashioned medical doctors point a shaming finger at women when they have PID because the stigma used to be, and still is with many doctors, that it is only caused by STD or Sexually Transmitted Diseases, numerous sexual partners and basically you're a whore. Of course this is not true. There are many causes for PID. Yes, sexually transmitted diseases are a big culprit, but we are not just talking about syphilis and gonorrhea. There is an almost endless amount of bacteria, fungus (yeast), and even virus that can cause PID. Gonorrhea is considered a major cause, but so is fungus or yeast, and there are over 15 different known types of trachomatis causing chlamydial infections. And 50% of women with these infections don't even know they have them. They are asymptomatic.

But besides the almost infinite micro-organisms that can cause PID and vaginal infections, there is healthy "good" bacteria that live there, too, similar to the healthy bacteria in your colon. These bacteria micro-flora protect your female organs and keep them healthy and strong. Spermicidal chemical creams and contraceptives and even condoms treated with chemicals, tampons with their bleaching and toxic chemicals, and the numerous female sprays and douches, even panty hose, antibiotics, etc. can also kill these friendly bacteria, causing these organs to lose their defensive ability and their friendly protective bacteria. Often vaginal overgrowth of Candida Albicans follows taking antibiotics just like it does in the colon. So here is the dilemma. Condoms and creams can prevent the cause of PID and vaginal infections, and antibiotics can treat them, but both can cause PID and vaginal infections, too. One natural safeguard is to have sexual intercourse only with healthy people. Although some may feel that this solution is too simple and innocent, it is actually almost foolproof if practiced diligently. Throughout my life I have made it a practice not to kiss girls who eat hamburgers and junk food, smoke cigarettes, and have a bad attitude, let alone have sexual intercourse with them. I have always kept my circle of sexual partners to people who frequent organic produce markets, health food stores, health retreats, fitness classes and vegetarian gatherings. In the dating before intercourse, whether it is an hour or a year, you can get a pretty good sense of a prospective partner's health level, if she smokes, bad habits, sexual history, etc. My sexual partners have to smell good and taste good, just like my food. Teaching my patients how to recognize healthy people and avoid the physically, emotionally and spiritually plagued kept them from attracting sexually transmitted diseases and infections far better than condoms and poison creams. For my patients that already had infections, I used the following routine.

DR. SCHULZE'S HERBAL FEMININE DOUCHE RECIPE

32 ounces of warm distilled water

the juice of half of an organic lemon

2 tablespoons of organic unfiltered raw apple cider vinegar

2 droppers-full of Echinacea Plus

1 dropper-full of Anti-Infection Formula

Chapter Seven

How To Improve the Quality of Your Life

THE LAW OF DIMINISHING RETURNS

Dr. Richard Schulze wrote in one of his bi-monthly newsletters the following:

"The United States lost again for the country with the longest life expectancy, and Japan won again. We didn't even make it into the top ten, not even close. Numerous countries all over the world have longer life spans and are outliving us like Greece, Spain, Israel, Sweden, Holland, even Iceland, the list is long. We did make the top ten on something though, i.e. countries that spend the most on medical care. Unfortunately we rank number one in the world. Interestingly enough, none of the countries listed above where people lived the longest were in the top ten of money spent on medical care. THIS PROVES WITHOUT A DOUBT THAT MEDICINE IS DEFINITELY A CASE OF THE MORE THAT YOU SPEND, THE LESS YOU GET!

JUST SAY NO TO DRUGS!

Our kids don't stand a chance anymore, not from the pushers that lurk in the alleys around school yards, but from the pushers inside the schools, the school nurses. Yes, in thousands of schools all across America, nurses are pushing drug carts from classroom to classroom with paper cups filled with pills, just like in the hospital, to medicate our supposedly misbehaved children.

In my clinic, hundreds of my patients' children were sent by their teachers to medical doctors to put them on powerful psychiatric and mood altering drugs. I would read the teachers reports of the children's horrendous crimes of daydreaming, having a vivid imagination, touching the other kids, singing, laughing, wiggling, doodling, hugging too much, having too much fun, and even praying. Have you ever noticed that these are all the same great traits we adults are now paying our good money to take classes, trying to relearn. Now in the new millennium, Fortune 500 companies are sending their top executives on vision quests and self expression seminars, in hopes to undo their frozen unimaginative minds, to develop new innovative products and new ways of doing business, while at the same time their kids are having their imagination drugged out of them in school. This is insane.

For most of us, the school system destroyed our sense of freedom, imagination, spontaneity, love and laughter and filled us with fear, anxiety, insecurity and self-doubt. It turned us into a race of followers, who don't dare to color outside the lines, rarely disagree with anyone, never question authority, follow the status quo, follow the rules and behave like good little boys and girls.

In my day, they just scared, intimidated, threatened and occasionally beat us into submission. But today, powerful chemical mind-zapping drugs are being used by dysfunctional school systems and bad, lazy teachers in overcrowded classrooms to get all the kids to come to attention, line up, shut up, do as you're told, and learn. I have taught for over 20 years all over the world, and call me old fashioned, but I thought the best way to get a student's attention was to be personally excited, passionate and involved in the subject, and figure out ways to get the students excited, having fun and involved too.

Check it out yourself, almost every murdering kid, from the Columbine High School murders, to the numerous other school shootings, to even that boy who raped, sodomized and then drowned that little girl face first in the toilet of a Nevada casino, was on mood altering medical doctor prescribed, teacher requested, pharmaceutical drugs. The press is too damned scared to talk about this one, I think because so many adults today are on Prozac, other anti-depressants and mood altering drugs, and hundreds of thousands of our kids are on them too. The problem is of such magnitude that it scares the hell out of people, so we pretend it doesn't exist. The only solution would be for people to take responsibility for themselves and their families and God only knows we are too busy to do that.

Ritalin and other drugs of this nature are known to backfire when the kid is agitated and pushed too far and have been proven to cause abnormal behavior all the way to frank psychotic episodes (disturbances of such magnitude that there is personality disintegration and loss of contact with reality), I would say that our kids who are assaulting, sodomizing, raping and murdering their classmates, have definitely had personality disintegration and lost contact with reality. Some don't even remember what they did when they are taken off the drugs.

A dear friend of mine told me last week that his wonderful kid was just prescribed Ritalin because the teacher said he looked at the classroom door and lost his attention when another kid walked through it, he was distracted. I said thank God the kid was alert since nowadays that classmate coming through the door could be some pharmaceutical drug doped up, suicidal zombie with a pipe bomb.

Prozac is now a commonly prescribed drug for 2 and 3 year old children who medical doctors, day care workers and nursery school teachers believe need to be psychologically altered.

We are all born geniuses, and some of us get less damaged then others as we grow up.

AM I TOO AGGRESSIVE?

Recently, I had some friends over to my house. They brought a man with them that I didn't know and he said to me that he thought that my newsletter, especially my Politically Incorrect column, was too aggressive, and that I was exhibiting too much rage. He said that I needed to be more loving. (He was referring to my attacks against medical doctors and the pharmaceutical industry, the biggest murderers and the #1 cause of death in America today, in my January 2000 Get Well Newsletter.)

Ironically this man's visit was cut short because his mother, who recently had breast cancer and had one breast hacked off by a doctor, was now having the other healthy breast ripped off her body, as some medically sick and perverted Frankenstein-ish idea of prevention. To this man, I guess that ignorant medical doctor cutting healthy tissue and body parts off his mother, supporting and promoting her to live in fear and ignorance, not teaching her about health and healing her body and ripping her off for thousands of dollars to torture her is O.K. or acceptable behavior. We should just smile? Say nothing? Be loving? Take our medicine? And that I, not the doctors, am the one who is out of control, acting inappropriate, too aggressive? NOW HOLD IT ONE DAMN MINUTE!

Have we become such ignorant, wimpy, gutless and spineless sheep, being led to the slaughter with love in our hearts and smiles on our faces? What a wonderful hypnotic con job medicine has done on us... O.K. Maybe I'll try to be a little more smoochy, woochy, but this guy was asking the wrong doctor to back down. If that were my mom, I would have helped her to make a more rational, sane and healthy decision based on strength, not fear, and illumination, not ignorance. I would have taken her to organic produce markets, shown her health food stores and health books, bought her a juicer and had a wheat grass juice party with her and maybe even a garlic enema. Taught her about cleansing and detoxification, hot and cold showers, skin brushing, herbal poultices, massage, laughter, and helped to educate her doctor and told him to shove the scalpel up his ass, in a positive, loving way of course.

The reality of medicine, all the pain, torture and disfigurement, is so horrible, the only way we can deal with it is to hide the truth, bury our heads in the sand, become numb and pretend it is a logical health care choice. Then when I illuminate the horror, and expose medicine for the criminally insane butchering and murder that it is, when people first see this, their first knee jerk reaction is to hate me, to kill the messenger. I know I push buttons, but never mistake that it is love and illumination, not anger and rage.

WHAT DO PAIN RELIEF, LIVER DEATH, AND THE MOVIE 'THE FUGITIVE' ALL HAVE IN COMMON?

Although many street drugs are toxic to your liver, the bigger danger is actually pharmaceutical drugs. You would also think that the big liver killers are the strong prescription drugs, but wrong again, some over the counter drugs are the biggest liver killers. Common aspirin substitute, over the counter pain relievers such as acetaminophin drugs cause Acute = SUDDEN, Hepatocellular = LIVER CELL and Necrosis = DEATH... meaning SUDDEN LIVER CELL DEATH!

How could this be? How could the FDA let this happen? Drugs are very strong chemicals, definitely NOT NATURAL SUBSTANCES and the liver tried like heck to get them out of your body. In its effort, it often hemorrhages, bleeds and dies and sometimes you die.

Remember the movie 'The Fugitive' with Harrison Ford and Tommy Lee Jones? Rent a copy, watch it and read behind the scenes of what is really going on. The whole reason why Dr. Kimball's wife was murdered and he was framed for it and imprisoned was because he was going to blow the whistle on a pharmaceutical company whose newest wonder drug was also killing liver cells and causing the liver to hemorrhage and people were dying. When he was going to expose that the drug was killing people, they tried to kill him instead. Hollywood does mimic life.

THE LIVER

Although your medical doctor would like for you to believe that he has figured your liver out and got it all down, the reality is that your liver is the most metabolically complex organ in the entire human body, more even than your brain. It has numerous different microscopic functional units and is as complex and infinite as outer space. One of the main reasons I know God was a natural healer and NOT a medical doctor is the liver itself. It is so incredibly complex, you know it is best to just leave it alone and create a lifestyle for it, and DON'T TOUCH IT, HANDS OFF. Now let me try to boil it down and make understanding the functions of the liver as simple as possible.

Your liver is the largest organ inside of your body. It weighs around 3 pounds. It is on your right side under your lower ribs. The underneath of your liver is concave because it covers your stomach, duodenum, hepatic flexure of the colon, right kidney and right adrenal. Blood passes through your liver, especially blood from your digestive organs, which contains end products of digestion and nutrition, before this blood enters your general circulation to the rest of your body. If I were to divide the two main tasks of your liver up, they would be ENERGY AND NUTRITION, and DETOXIFICATION.

ENERGY AND NUTRITION

Your liver is your life force, the source for your energy. Your liver synthesizes the sugar glucose from carbohydrates or starches that you eat. Glucose is the most important carbohydrate in your body's metabolism. It could just be called PURE ENERGY because it is used by your brain and every other cell of the body and for just that, energy.

Excess glucose is stored in your liver as glycogen and is ready to be converted back to glucose if any energy is needed. Your liver also stores other super energy nutrients like vitamin B-12 and iron to be used anytime you need a turbo charge.

Your liver also makes vitamins, clotting factors and amino acids. It makes cholesterol that you need to produce steroid hormones (sex hormones) and other important metabolic chemicals. It also makes the lipoproteins like HDLs that transport fat around in your blood. (If you have too much cholesterol in your blood causing coronary arterial blockages, this is caused from eating too much animal food and rarely from a liver gone haywire.) The liver stores other vitamins like A, D, E and K.

DETOXIFICATION

Your liver is the blood detoxification organ of your body. The liver recycles and removes worn out blood cells.

Each red blood cell has a life span of 120 days (4 months). Once it is too old and its time is up, macrophanges, big eating white blood cells in your liver eat them. Every RBC (red blood cell) contains hemoglobin. Hemoglobin is the iron containing pigment in your blood that makes it red, which carries the oxygen from your lungs to all the cells in your body. Your liver recycles this iron, stores it for later use, or turns it into bile which it excretes and is a digestive juice.

Bile stimulates digestion, emulsifies fats, stimulates peristalsis (the muscular waves of the intestines), and is a natural laxative and a natural digestive antiseptic.

Bile contains bilirubin, a yellow-orange pigment from the iron in the hemoglobin from the dead red blood cells that macrophanges ate… phew, if you didn't catch that one don't worry, remember getting well is easy.

NOW FOR THE NUMBER FREAKS

Each red blood cell has over 200 million hemoglobin molecules in it and you have over 35 trillion red blood cells, so that's over 7,000,000,000,000,000,000 (how do you say this number?) hemoglobin molecules that your liver has to recycle or over 58,000,000,000,000 (58 trillion) hemoglobin molecules every day. O.K. let's get simple. The liver detoxifies, metabolizes, renders harmless and eliminates harmful toxic poisons, chemicals, and substances from your blood. It produces many different enzymes that actually convert toxic poisons into harmless chemicals and then they are eliminated in the bile that your liver excretes.

A small list of substances that your liver detoxifies and renders harmless are alcoholic drinks, street drugs, pharmaceutical drugs, insecticides, pesticides, food additives, environmental toxic chemicals, parasites, bacteria and virus. So one of the liver's main jobs is to eliminate toxins, chemicals, poisons and drugs from your body. Then it only makes sense that the more intake you have of toxic substances, the harder it is on your liver, the more work it has to do. This makes a great case for organic food, it not only tastes better and is more nutritious, but it doesn't overwork or deplete your liver.

The liver also has to metabolize and render harmless anything that causes increased ammonia in the body. The main culprit here is animal food. When animal food is digested, it forms ammonia, an alkaline gas, which is absorbed by your intestines into your blood to be hopefully converted into urea by your liver to be removed by your kidneys. Americans being the highest consumers of animal food on the planet per person, have a constant over production of ammonia gas in the intestines which in turn weakens the liver and promotes hepatic coma or paralysis of the liver. Substances that contain ammonia, besides animal flesh, organs, eggs and milk, are mainly drugs such as sedatives, tranquilizers, anesthetics, analgesics (pain relievers) and diuretics. (AT HOME EXPERIMENT: Take two aspirin and place them in a spoon over a candle or a stove until the aspirin melt, WOW, ammonia city.) For years in my clinic, I saw patient after patient with liver trauma and even acute failure that causes hepatic coma worse than alcohol, drugs and toxic poisons. IT WAS CAUSED BY FAD HIGH PROTEIN DIETS. These diets have come and gone and current ones are the Zone and the Atkins. These diets, like any diet, can cause weight loss, but they can also skyrocket your ammonia levels and paralyze your liver. This is a double whammy because your liver now cannot process all this added cholesterol that you are eating more and more of, and this alone could give you a heart attack or stroke. Granted you will look fit and trim in the hospital bed or the casket, but better to have a healthy liver than to be sick or dead.

WHEN YOUR LIVER GETS SICK

One of your liver's primary jobs is the production of bile, which is its waste product and also a great digestive system amongst many other things. When the liver gets sick, it gets constipated and the bile, instead of getting released, backs up in the body.

Remember the part before about the 58 trillion hemoglobin molecules that the liver has to process EVERY DAY from the dead red blood cells. Well if the liver backs up with bile which contains bilirubin, an orange-red iron pigment from the old hemoglobin that the liver eats, and at the same time the liver also can't continue to clean all the 58 trillion a day recently dead orange-red hemoglobin molecules out of your blood, well in a very short time have all this excess circulating orange-red bilirubin and hemoglobin and what color do you think you are going to turn, you guessed it, ORANGE-RED. When your sclera (the whites of your eyes), your skin and even your urine takes on an orange-red color, this is called jaundice and is a good sign that your liver is very constipated, it is that simple. This is why one of the major cleansing and detoxifying aids I used in my clinic was a silver flush, to unconstipate the liver and get the bile flowing again. There are two major types of jaundice and they are referred to as Intra Hepatic, (inside your liver), and Extra Hepatic (outside of your liver) that refer to where it is thought the trouble is.

INTRA HEPATIC JAUNDICE

The most common causes of hepatitis (which just means liver inflammation) and Intra Hepatic Jaundice are drugs, alcohol, liver damage, almost any virus, bacteria, fungus, fad heavy animal protein weight loss diets, and viral hepatitis.

VIRAL HEPATITIS

There are currently 6 known types of viral hepatitis. The most commonly known are Hepatitis A, Hepatitis B and what used to be referred to as Hepatitis non-A, non-B, which is now called Hepatitis C, and Hepatitis D, E, and G. Soon we will discover so many more that we will run out of letters of the alphabet and have to start giving them names like tropical storms and hurricanes, like Hepatitis Harry. All through the current medical mass panic is to vaccinate for Hepatitis C and the vaccination is given to 1 day old children in NYC and most school kids in California, the only real prevention is to STOP doing what hurts your liver, like drugs and toxins, and START living a healthy liver lifestyle. As I said earlier, the liver's job is to neutralize poisons and toxins, and the more a person is bombarded with poisons, the weaker the liver becomes. What poisons you ask, well when was the last time you were around a typical American kid, and watched him eat, or any adult for that matter. Weak livers have less resistance to infections. We will never get rid of germs and virus, as I always say the only defense is a strong offense, building a strong healthy body. The massive amount of hepatitis infections all around America is just a reflection that we have beaten up our livers for too long.

EXTRA HEPATIC JAUNDICE

The most common cause of Extra Hepatic Jaundice is some type of blockage, sounds like my theory of all disease caused by blockage, doesn't it, and the major blockage is gall stones stuck in the gall bladder and bile ducts. Remember I said earlier that over half a million people this year in America will have their gall bladders carved out of them by medical doctors. Medical doctors are so absolutely stupid, FLUSH IT OUT, don't CUT IT OUT.

Minor jaundice or liver constipation can go on for years almost unnoticed, causing all sorts of health related problems. Neurological diseases, Neuromuscular diseases, paralysis, chronic fatigue, immune system depression, and disorders, cancer, heart disease, stroke, hypertension, high cholesterol, every digestive disorder from indigestion to constipation, diabetes, dementia, depression, painful and stiff joints, sexual dysfunction, eyesight problems, the list is almost endless.

Many old age doctors used to say when you have someone that has cancer, you have a patients who had a sick liver 3 to 5 years ago. I will go a step further, with any sick patient and with any disease, we need to look at the liver and get it clean. That is why in my clinic, EVERYONE, EVERY PATIENT had to do my 5 day cleansing and detoxification program and my liver and gall bladder flush. What is the bottom line? Let the liver get run down and congested and you will become toxic and weak. Keep the liver healthy and you will be protected from chemical poisons, disease, feel great and have tons of energy.

THE GALLBLADDER

The gallbladder is a pear shaped sac on the underside of the right lobe of the liver that stores bile from the liver. While in the gallbladder, the bile is concentrated by removing the water. The bile is released through the cystic duct, which joins the hepatic duct from the liver to create the common bile duct which empties into the duodenum (the beginning of the small intestine). Bile is not only the waste product of the liver that carries away the neutralized poisons, but as stated previously, also stimulates digestion, aids digestion by emulsifying fats, stimulates peristalsis (the muscular waves of the intestines), is a natural laxative and a natural digestive antiseptic.

When the bile contains too much cholesterol from eating too much animal food, or for some people ANY animal food, the cholesterol can't be kept in solution any more and forms quite hard stones and rocks. These can form in the gallbladder and also the bile ducts causing Extra Hepatic Jaundice. (Use Dr. Schulze's Liver Gallbladder Flush to get rid of your rock collection.)

THE LIVER FLUSH
AND WHAT IT DOES

(This is part of Dr. Schulze's 5 day Cleansing and Detoxification Program.) The main cause of liver and gallbladder disease is an overworked liver that is overloaded with toxins and poisons from our food, water and air and also from taking drugs, drinking alcohol and eating too much animal food. All of these cause the liver and gall bladder to be overloaded and subsequently congest, get constipated and you get sick. This is the cause of many seemingly unrelated diseases, EVEN CANCER, and these are the things that you need to STOP.

The liver and gallbladder flush drink and herbal formula stimulate the liver to produce more bile and get the bile moving through the gallbladder and ducts. This action unblocks and unconstipates the liver and gallbladder and even dissolves and removes gallstones. This is what will clean, detoxify, and heal your liver and gallbladder and what you need to start.

NOTE BY AUTHOR: You may get the 5 day Cleansing and Detoxification Program by contacting Dr. Schulze's business office at 1-800-HERBDOC.

In addition, be sure to review Chapter 23 to see another idea how you may add 10-15 years to your life and feel better during the rest of your life.

Chapter Eight

There IS a Cure for the Common Cold

The average American gets infected with numerous bacterial and viral pathogens every winter and gets 3 to 4 colds lasting between 2 and 3 weeks each. Most people believe this pain and suffering is just "the way it is" and is unavoidable. After all, even our top medical doctors tell us there is no cure for the common cold.

On the contrary, the average patient in my clinic that followed my programs did not get sick every winter. In fact they stayed cold and flu free for years, even decades! They did this by creating strong powerful immune systems that destroyed and killed harmful micro-organisms before they had a chance to dig in. And for those new patients who walked into my clinic already infected with a cold or flu, I taught them natural programs that annihilated cold and flu infections within 24 to 48 hours.

So you can imagine my horror when I heard people say that natural treatments and herbs for colds and flu don't work! When I heard people say that, I'll be honest, it pissed me off, that is, until I realized that they were right!

Don't be surprised, they are right, because the natural cold and flu prevention programs I see in magazines, books and health food stores couldn't possibly work. At best they are wimpy and weak programs that might possibly maybe kind-of soothe scratchy throats and slightly ease your sniffles. And if you think that impotent, invisible homeopathic duck-liver crap, or the watered down herbal junk out there will save you...well, you are in for a BIG disappointment. Bacteria and Virus eat wimpy, weak and watered-down for breakfast. You screw around with pathogenic killer micro-organisms and you can die. So what do you do? KILL THEM AND KILL THEM DEAD! In my clinic, I learned the hard way that this is all out war! I had to watch a few of my patients die before I figured out that I had to turn the intensity and volume way up with my healing programs and herbal dosages, especially when it came to treating colds and influenza. When it comes to bacterial and viral infections, you have to kick their ass before they kick yours. There is no time to waste. These are bacterial and viral terrorists, their bodies wrapped in TNT and their car trunks are packed with C4 explosives, and they are driving right at you... a hundred miles an hour, and they want you DEAD. You screw around, waste time, wimp out, hesitate... you die.

I used two programs in my clinic. The first, prevention, isn't a strong enough word for what I am going to show you. The second program, in case you already have a cold or flu, is an all out natural blitzkrieg against the invaders. Doses of Echinacea and Garlic so high even the toughest herbalists faint, and hydrotherapy and diaphoretic routines so powerful they could drive the devil itself out of your body.

What's the bottom line? Somebody is going to suffer and die... and with my programs, I make damn sure it's them and not you.

"Why does cold and flu season happen only during the winter months? How can you tell when it's starting and how do I get myself and my family prepared?"

Generally cold and flu season starts in September or October, and it ends in March or April. That's a standard for most areas in the Northern Hemisphere. One of the ways that you can almost always tell, whatever part of the country that you live in, is when you start turning the heating on in the house. I remember as a kid, my dad used to put the storm windows up, the extra-insulated windows that you don't see as much of anymore. It's the time of year when all of a sudden it gets colder at night. It might even still be hot during the day, but it gets colder at night, and then eventually, usually within a week or so, it gets cold during the day also. That's when you know it's the beginning of the cold and flu season. Now that I've said that, there are influenzas that come around in the summertime, too. But generally speaking it starts in September-October and runs through to March and April.

"But how does that cause colds and flu?"

It's very simple. People are closer to each other, breathing less fresh air. During the winter months, when we shut the windows of the house more, we have less fresh air coming in, and when people are inside they spread disease from one person to another because of our confinement- breathing the same air and being in close proximity with other people without the fresh air. Just like going into an airplane: your chances of getting an infection are much greater when you go into an airplane versus if you just walk down the road, and it's simply because the air is being re-circulated and you're breathing the same air in a more concentrated way that the other people are exhaling. So if one person or two people get on a plane and they're sick, there's a much greater chance that everyone else on board is going to get the same illness. Or in an office building that doesn't have fresh air, doesn't re-circulate the air... the same thing. So this time of the year we're breathing a greater concentration of other people's air, and of course if anybody is sneezing or coughing, we're breathing the air from that person that's contaminated with bacteria or a virus. So that's why it happens this time of year.

One of the greatest ways you can prevent getting a cold or flu is not putting yourself in a situation like that. Travel less on airplanes this time of year. If you do travel on airplanes, wear a facemask. You might look a little strange or some people might think you're in the Michael Jackson club, but it's not a bad idea. If you're afraid of looking that strange, I have a lot of patients and customers who used to just take some type of cotton cloth or a paper towel and spray it with Clinical Air therapy and keep that near their mouth and breathe through that. Of course, that kills bacteria and virus. And also, you're kind of filtering the air you breathe through a solution that is known to kill bacteria and virus. So try not to put yourself in these situations. I know some people have to work in an office. See if you can get out and get some fresh air a couple times a day. And also prevention, the minute you notice people getting sick whether it's an airplane or in your office, that's the time to start my Preventative Program that we'll talk about in a little bit.

"I get sick all the time. I get sick when the seasons change, I get sick when I work too much, and if anybody around me gets sick, I get sick too. What can I do to keep myself from getting sick all the time?"

First of all, you should acknowledge that this is your greatest blessing from God that you get sick all the time. I know this might be hard to understand at first, but give me a minute. You have inherited a weak constitution, and everybody inherits weak things in their constitution from their parents. And yours seems to be your immune strength. If you did not inherit a weak immune system from your parents, and you have a good or normal or strong immune system, then your lifestyle is so horrendous that it's weakening your immune system. It can only be one or the other. But if you find yourself, like some people, constantly getting colds and flu and sick all the time, you either inherited a weak immune system or you have a lifestyle that's destroying your immune system, or both. Now, the reason I say that this is a blessing is because this is a monitor. I can help you create a lifestyle where you never get sick. And then you'll know you've done what's necessary to either boost up your lifestyle so your weakened immune system constitution doesn't affect you, or to change your lifestyle to where you don't degrade your immune system. So the simple answer for a person who gets sick all the time is you need to be healthy. I know this might sound overly simple, or redundant, but this is the type of person who needs to increase their level of health, and if you do that enough you'll get to a point where you never, ever, ever get sick. So the first step is you want to create a healthier lifestyle. You need to eliminate the foods that you're eating that degrade your immune system or make it hard on your immune system, especially animal foods. Imagine the amount of bacteria and harmful pathogenic micro-organisms that are in dead animal flesh. No matter how much you cook it, they're still there. So this type person needs to become a vegan vegetarian. Stop eating all bacteria-laden animal products and milk and dairy and eggs. Get on a nice healthy vegetarian food program. This person needs to do all my routine cleanses from the Bowel Cleanse first, to the Liver and Gallbladder Cleanse, and then to the Kidney and Bladder Cleanse. This person needs to be living on SuperFood and getting the nutrition in, and do all my foundational health and healing programs. This person will find that after about a 6 month period of taking care of themselves, they'll stop getting sick. This is simply a sign that you're not well, and either your immune system you inherited is not strong enough to take care of you, or your lifestyle is degraded enough to where it's keeping your immune system weak. Often this type of person will say something like, but I do exactly what Jane does who sits at the desk next to me, or I do exactly what my friend Harry does but he's never sick. Well, you're not your friend Harry, you're not your friend Jane, you are not your co-workers. You are like a fingerprint, a snowflake, an individual with different parents, and you cannot do exactly the same as the person next to you and expect the same results. If you're sick all the time, you need to clean up your lifestyle and strengthen your immune system.

"My six-year-old boy, even though he's healthy, doesn't have a very good constitution. He has constant bouts with asthma, and every once in a while he gets a respiratory infection combined with a fever. The fever gets as high as a hundred and four degrees. I know you are a parent, so I know you'll understand when I say it's frightening. What can I do to keep him from getting sick this season?"

I am a parent, and I know exactly what you mean. For any parent, even the great Dr. Schulze, you feel a bit helpless when your children are sick and you would gladly cut a finger off if that would help them get well immediately. But that's the blessing of natural healing: you can't heal anybody- people have to heal themselves. And the way that you're going to keep your child from getting sick all the time is with a great dose of common sense. The first thing that I know when I hear about a kid who has bouts with asthma and coughs and colds and respiratory infections all the time is you have to get off all dairy products. Dairy products are the great congesters of the lungs. You might think 'well, I don't know if my kid is lactose intolerant?' Every human is lactose intolerant to cow's milk. Cow's milk is not a natural food for the human body. It's the beautiful food with all the fats and hormones FOR A COW. Humans are only designed to have human milk, and only up until they cut their teeth, or about a year and a half, to two years of age, is the necessity. So one of the first signs of lactose intolerance in kids is the congestion in the sinuses and the lungs. So you need to stop dairy products immediately, put that kid on a vegan food program, get the juicer out and get the nutrition into that kid with the juicer and SuperFood, and you're going to notice a huge difference right away. And I haven't even started with building his immunity with Echinacea Plus. And remember, you mentioned the kid gets a high fever… the fever is the friend. It removes the garbage from the body. It gets all the pathogenic micro-organisms out of your system, the bacteria, the virus, whatever. So keep the kid hydrated during the fever, lots and lots and lots of liquid. Distilled water, fresh juices… and to keep your kid from getting sick this season, get on that good food program, build that kid a strong, healthy constitution, and do my Prevention and Treatment Programs outlined in this newsletter. Depending on the age of your child, children can take the standard Echinacea Plus or they can take the children's formula. But if your child is eight or nine years of age, you can move on the Echinacea Plus.

I am amazed at how parents lose their consciousness when it comes to their children and don't modify their food programs, still give them treats when they are sick, from chocolate and sodas to dairy products and all the garbage. It's very important for a parent to not lose their consciousness when their child is sick and get them on a good food program immediately. Even a day or two of a juice fast is OK. Children will naturally lose their appetite when they're not feeling well, so parents, be strong and get your kids well and get them on the programs.

"I just found out I'm pregnant and my doctor is strongly recommending I get a flu shot. I absolutely hate that stuff and don't want to do it, but if I get sick, I'm scared for the baby. What can I do?"

Did you know that recently, Dr. J. Anthony Morris, former Chief Vaccine Control Officer at the FDA, stated, "There is no evidence that any influenza vaccine thus far developed is effective in preventing or mitigating any attack of influenza. The producers of these vaccines know that they are worthless, but they go on selling them anyway."

You don't even have a child and you're already in the first steps of parent hell. The reality is that as a parent you will have to make numerous decisions that can affect the life of your child. In fact, some of them may even be life or death decisions. Because after the flu shot is going to come inoculations for your baby. And a hundred other questions... what do you do? They could die from the inoculations. They could die from an infection they get. The reality is you're asking me, and I'm a naturopath. I'm a natural healer, and I can't think of anything worse than when you're building a baby inside of your body that you would inject some of the most lethal garbage poison known to man. I would never suggest that a mother-to-be have any type of flu shot. The outcome can be horrendous, even lethal. Do not put that type of poison into your body. The best way to make sure that you do not get the flu is to do something proactive, like my Prevention Program. Make sure that you do it every month. My strong advice on the flu shot: don't do it. On the other hand, herbs when you are pregnant are fine. All of my programs can be done while you are pregnant. You just have to use your good common sense and don't do anything too abrupt or harsh, especially during the last trimester. But there isn't an herbal product that I have that you can't use from the beginning of your pregnancy to the end of your pregnancy. Again, just use your good common sense.

"I know I've heard you say that antibiotics are bad. I also know that the flu car kill people. So if antibiotics kill the flu, how can they be so bad?"

First of all, antibiotics don't kill the flu, they don't work against the flu at all! According to the AMA, and most medical experts, antibiotics are absolutely USELESS for colds, influenza and upper respiratory tract infections. They have no preventative nor curing effect on influenza even though American medical doctors this year will write millions and millions of prescriptions for them to their patients with the flu. According to Fred Rubin, MD, associate clinical professor of medicine at the University of Pittsburgh and contributor to the Merck Manual- Home Edition, "Not only are antibiotics powerless against the viruses that cause colds and flu, but misuse of antibiotics can actually do more harm than good." According to the Journal of the American Medical Association, the high rates of antibiotic prescribing and misuse has caused alarming increases in new harmful drug resistant organisms.

And as far as getting a flu vaccine shot, did you know, if you had five consecutive flu shots in any decade your chances of getting Alzheimer's Disease is TEN TIMES HIGHER. This is partially due to the mercury and aluminum that is in every flu shot (and most childhood shots) that builds up in the brain and causes cognitive dysfunction and disease. This is partially why the rate of Alzheimer's Disease is skyrocketing.

Remember what I always say- Drugs don't EDUCATE your immune system. Killing diseases with harsh and dangerous chemical drugs at best is only a temporary quick fix. Your immune system is left uneducated so the same disease will return again, and usually with a vengeance the second time around. This is why people who try to kill a cold or flu with drugs usually have constant recurring colds and flu. This is also why after a medical doctor cuts, burns or poisons out a person's cancer, it almost always returns. The body and immune system were never educated, no real healing took place, only part of a disease was killed and the person is still living a cold, flu or even cancer creating lifestyle. The disease, just like Arnold in The Terminator, says "I'll be back," because not only do drugs only kill part of the disease, and the leftover parts become stronger and are more drug resistant, but also you didn't do anything to stop creating more disease.

Curing diseases with a healthy lifestyle creates a strong and educated immune system so you don't have a recurrence of the same problem later. Your body was supported with great nutrition and cleansing and it figured out how to HEAL you all by itself. THIS IS THE ONLY TRUE HEALING, SELF HEALING. Diseases are the by-product of a faulty lifestyle, therefore the only real cure, the only real healing for anything, is creating a healthier lifestyle and letting your body heal you.

The only true healing or cure for ANYTHING, but especially the common cold, is the one your body can create by living a healthy lifestyle. Your body can heal itself of ANYTHING; all it needs is your help. Living a healthy lifestyle will also prevent future disease before it even starts by building you a strong and powerful, protective, immune system.

"I've heard you say a person can stop a cold or flu dead in it's tracks naturally. So what do I do when I go to bed with a sore throat, hoping it will go away during the night, and wake up with it flaring?"

One of the first things that I have my patients do, and certainly the first thing that I do at any sign of some type of bacterial viral infection, which could be a fever, sore throat, congested sinuses, congested lungs, whatever, is I take a high dose of Echinacea and SuperTonic. Which would be 1 to 2 ounces of Echinacea Plus and a ½ ounce to 1 ounce of SuperTonic. Mix these herbal tonics with 16 ounces of a water/juice combination. This can be drunk all at once or over a period of a few hours before bed.

The second thing is take that bath, my Cold and Flu-busting Hydrotherapy Bath. So imagine now you have 1 to 2 ounces of Echinacea, a half ounce of SuperTonic, say you have that in about 16 ounces of liquid. Also get some hot tea going, peppermint, ginger, throw a little cayenne with the Echinacea and a little juice, and get in that hot bath and follow the hot bath routine as follows.

Turn on the heater in the bathroom and get the room as hot as you can. Run a hot bath as hot as you can stand it. Add some sea salt, bath salts or seaweed if you have it. Once you are in, if you can stand it, add more hot water and increase the temperature even more.

While you are in the tub drink at least 6 cups of herbal tea. A Ginger root and Peppermint leaf blend is one of my favorites, but even hot water with a little lemon juice and cayenne pepper will do. Make it palatable and warm (not hot) because you want to drink at least 6 cups in the next 15 to 20 minutes.

You will begin to sweat, stay in as long as you can- at least 20 minutes. If at anytime during this routine you feel faint, put a cold washcloth or your face and put some cayenne tincture or cayenne pepper in your mouth. Rinse off cool, dress warm and go to bed. You will wake up in the morning without your cold and flu and feel like a million bucks.

"How do you suggest to consume raw garlic?"

There are a couple of ways. One way, if you feel like you can't tolerate it very well as far as the burning in your mouth or the intensity of the garlic, is to chop it up and put it in a spoon and just put it in your mouth and knock it back and swallow it with some liquid. The important part about chopping it up is the garlic has two cells in it, a fiber cell and a liquid cell, and the potent antibacterial aspect of garlic is the allicin, and allicin is only created when you chop, grind, pound, or break up the garlic. So it's important to chop it up and not swallow the cloves whole. So chop it up and spoon it down and swallow it. If you have a sensitive stomach you might want to buffer your stomach a little bit with just a little liquid or possibly having it with dinner. If it's around dinner time and you have a little food in your stomach, start consuming some raw garlic, a lot of raw garlic. When I talk about raw garlic, I usually only talk in amounts of 10 or 20 cloves. So consume a tremendous amount of raw garlic with your dinner.

"I've heard from friends that take your products that you don't believe the old saying 'feed a cold and starve a fever, I'm confused."

Or was it 'feed a fever and starve a cold'? Anyway, it doesn't matter what your grandmother told you, because the answer is STARVE EVERYTHING! Anytime you feel the first signs of anything coming on, STOP EATING and FLUSH your body out with pure water, herb tea and fresh juices. My purifying, immune-building Food Program is STEP 1.

It takes a lot of energy to process, digest, assimilate and eliminate food. If you continue to eat while having a purification it is harder for your body to heal. If you stop eating, your body can utilize ALL of its energy and resources to help you get well. Juices are the concentrated liquid extracts of food. This means they can be digested with very little effort and are concentrated sources of vitamins, minerals and other nutrients. Your body needs these nutrients to manufacture immune cells, rebuild immune organs, and create vital immune chemicals, like antibodies, that you need to destroy bacteria, virus or any pathogen. Some of these nutrients on their own, like vitamins A and C, have natural infection fighting and immune stimulating ability.

These juices also flush toxins and poisons out of the body and also naturally purge the body and open up the elimination organs. So stop eating and get the juicer out. Use local organic produce that is in season. You can dilute the juice with up to 50% water. For some this makes it easier to digest. You must consume at least one gallon (128 ounces) of fluid each day on this program. That can be a combination of fruit juice, vegetable juice, herb tea and pure water. Do Not Forget to take your SuperFood! And if you are sick, take it 2 times a day.

Consume at least 3 cloves of fresh RAW garlic each day. NO deodorized capsules. Garlic is a potent antiviral and antibacterial herb. It destroys both gram positive and gram negative bacteria. In other words it's an all-natural broad-spectrum antibiotic. But the best part is that unlike chemical antibiotic pills, Garlic leaves all of your friendly and good bacteria alone and alive, the bacteria that you need to be healthy. Pharmaceutical antibiotics are non-selective in their destruction of bacteria and destroy even your good bacteria. That is why you end up with digestive problems, constipation, and yeast and fungal overgrowth infections. Garlic, on the other hand, actually enhances your intestinal micro-flora and selectively kills the bad bacteria. Mother Nature does it best again!

"I've had some sort of flu for over a month now. I cough and I ache and my head throbs. No matter what I do, I can't seem to kick it. Every time I think it's going away, it comes back, sometimes even worse than before. How can I get rid of it and can I do it naturally?"

If you can't kick it, it's because you haven't been aggressive enough. Whenever any kind of disease remains in your body, it just means that you haven't stopped enough of the things that you're doing that make you sick and you haven't started doing enough of the things that will make you better. Or maybe you started doing enough of them, but you're not doing them intensely enough or aggressively enough. One of the reasons I became famous in my clinic for helping people heal themselves of diseases that other doctors couldn't do naturally is because I turned up the volume, the dosages, the intensity in which we do the routines. So this is what you are not doing. You need to take a look at my 7-Step program and do it aggressively. You need to get yourself well. Anybody that continues to have a cold or flu, it's a sign of a weak immune system, and it's a sign that you're still beating your immune system up with your lifestyle. And I would be concerned about a long-term cold or flu, but I would also be concerned about whatever diseases might be lurking in your body. The cold or flu might just be the tip of the iceberg. So this is a sign that a person is not healthy and it's time to really turn your life around and get on an aggressive health program.

"Every cold and flu season I come down with something. I know how to get better naturally in only a few days, but my cough always persists, sometimes for weeks. How do I get rid of the nagging cough?"

You know how to get rid of your cold and flu in only a few days-that's great! Pretty much everybody who follows my advice has learned how to do that. But if you have a nagging cough, you need a high dose over a period of one to two days where you're consuming at least an ounce, if not two ounces, of Echinacea Plus over the period of a day with ½ to 1 ounce of SuperTonic. You'll find that the cough will do away within a couple of days. And if you want to amp that up, use twenty cloves of garlic a day. A great herb for the bacteria that can be in the lungs. Just the odor as you breathe after eating garlic will disinfect the bacteria and virus, will kill the bacteria and virus in your lungs. Use my Echinacea Plus and SuperTonic and get to know and love garlic.

Chapter Nine

What About Success Stories? By Dr. Richard Schulze

Last fall I was sitting in my office reading a few of the literally thousands of letters I receive every year. Most of these letters are personal testimonials of people who have healed themselves of all types of Cancer, Heart Disease, Neurological and Muscular Diseases, Alzheimers, Diabetes, Arthritis… the list of diseases is almost endless.

At the same time a friend of mine called that was recently diagnosed with Pancreatic Cancer and was beginning my Incurables Program. When I was telling him about some of these healing miracle letters he asked me if I would let him call someone who has healed themselves of cancer using my programs. I told him NO, absolutely not!

The first reason I don't do that is because I take my patients' privacy very seriously. I remember during the peak years of my clinic I received many offers, even a few blank checks from scandal rags and star magazines, if I would just leave a patient file in my mailbox. I never did. I used to say that I don't know if the reason I am such a popular doctor with the entertainment community is because I am a great doctor, or just because I kept my mouth shut. But in any case, I never disclosed any information about any patient of mine, EVER!

I also never promoted my new patients talking to my long time patients for another reason. New patients like this man would often ask, "Can't I talk to someone who has healed themselves of my same disease?" On the very few occasions that I did introduce a new patient to long term patients who gave permission, the results never satisfied the new patients.

People with degenerative, serious and life-threatening diseases often want to find proof that Natural Healing and Herbal Medicine works, instead of just focusing on healing themselves. More often they just don't want proof, they want to find someone with their exact same disease that has healed themselves naturally.

But I found that most people who are in search for proof, even when they get it, are still not satisfied. They are like bottomless pits. Psychic Energetic Vampires.

The bottom line is that when you are told that you have cancer or some other life-threatening disease, most people go into a nose dive. Horribly frightened and having to make rushed life and death decisions for usually the first time in their lives, they feel their whole life falling apart and they often crash and burn. This is when they think that seeking out proof will help them, hoping to be convinced or, worse yet, trying to convince their medical doctors that there is another option besides chemotherapy, surgery, radiation or whatever.

On the few occasions that I would make the introduction, the new patient would almost always come back to me and say, "But their Leukemia is a little different type than mine." Even when I would find them a patient with the exact same disease, then they would say, "But I think mine is worse or more aggressive," or "Their tumor is smaller, or bigger, or a different type or color," or "I've had mine longer," or "They are a woman and I am a man," or "They don't have the same level of stress that I have had," or "as much responsibility," or "They are younger," or "stronger willed," or "I have much more to lose," or

"Let me see their blood tests," or "Let em see their tumor pathology report," or "Let me talk to their doctor," or "Let me talk to one more patient," or blah, blah, blah, blah, blah, blah and freaking more blah.

I Broke My Own Rules

Totally ignoring this experience, I believed that maybe this time, with my friend, it would be different. So after a few days I agreed to let my friend with pancreatic cancer call a few of the people who have written me letters, if it was OK with them. So I called my best friend and CEO of American Botanical Pharmacy, Adam Loef, and asked him if he would call a few of our customers who had sent healing miracle letters to me and ask them if they would mind receiving a call from my friend. Well, all of them, to my great surprise, said "have him call me right away!"

Another reason I thought this might work this time when it had failed in the past is because my friend with the cancer is a very smart man, and very successful in his business. He was not just successful at being healthy. So I figured a man this smart, one who has created so much, well, he must have a lot of great success tools. So if I can just get him to put half the energy he put into being a business success into being a healing success and healing his disease, well, I was sure he could heal himself in just a few months.

So I thought that maybe I would try one more time to see if anyone could ever get something out of talking to someone who had healed themselves. To my great surprise, HE DID!

But my friend, instead of searching for proof like some first year law student, was looking for something different. Actually, what he told me was he was just looking for some positive feedback because he got nothing positive from the medical doctors. He felt that if he could hear something positive and healing, instead of just negativity and killing disease, it would help him counteract the powerful, horrifying and very negative information that was circulating in his mind, that was told to him by some of the world's leading medical doctors.

He also told me this analogy. He said that when you grow a crystal on a string, the string must be dipped into a solution. But first you need a seed crystal on the string. What he realized was that he didn't have the seed crystal to heal himself. He needed to implant some healing seeds into his mind, the same way a farmer plants seeds into the ground.

I have always said that no farmer has ever planted strawberries and then found corn coming up in the field, you always get what you plant. You will harvest what you plant; you will reap what you sow. In other words, this man knew that tomorrow will be what he believes and does today and so he needed some different seeds, some healing seeds.

From the medical doctors he received disease, fear, horror and death seeds, but he wanted some love and healing seeds, some seeds that would tell him what is possible. He knew he needed to go to a different seed store. So instead of getting more seeds from medical doctors he decided to get some seeds from some of the customers of American Botanical Pharmacy.

My friend talked to a few of my customers who had written letters about their miracle healings. He said that he used talking to these people as a catalyst to lift himself up and begin his own personal healing experience.

After he talked with just two people, Martin from Florida and Toni Law from California, both of whom I have interviewed in this newsletter, I saw a huge and immediate shift in my friend. He changed dramatically, and for the first time I could hear some power in his voice, he was no longer the whining victim. He had now empowered himself and was well on his way to healing himself. It was just the right seed, the spark that he needed to ignite his own healing flame.

So it was at this moment last fall that I called back Adam Loef and told him that at American Botanical Pharmacy, that I was going to do a very rare thing. Maybe for the first time in decades, I was going to shut my mouth. I was going to let my customers and patients do the talking. People were told by their medical doctors that they would be dead years ago from their killer diseases, but they didn't die, they are very much alive. In fact, they are thriving and many have outlived the same medical doctors that gave them the death sentence. Use them as seeds to lift yourself up, to create a healthier life, to heal disease and to learn that there are many realities in life.

One is the medical reality, filled with pain, torture, disfigurement, drugs, sickness, horror, and fear. It will eat up your life savings in a heartbeat, and will ultimately kill you.

The other is Natural Healing and Herbal Medicine. It is the reality of Responsibility instead of blame, the reality of Simple instead of complicated, the reality of Change instead of stuck and, most important, it is the reality of assisting your body in its most primary function, Healing Itself instead of letting medical doctors try to cut, burn and poison you well. It is the reality that Tomorrow IS whatever you DO and BELIEVE Today, RIGHT NOW!

It is the reality of healing yourself of ANYTHING, ANY DISEASE! All you have to do is STOP doing what you did that made you sick in the first place and START doing some new things that will assist your body in doing what it was designed to do, HEAL ITSELF, AND HEAL YOU!

CANCER, CANCER

Just the word Cancer itself might be the most frightening word in the English language, in fact in ANY language. For most of my patients just the diagnosis of cancer turned them into helpless, sobbing incurable victims with thoughts of a mutilating alien disease spreading rapidly and uncontrollably through their body. This disease would destroy their family emotionally, spiritually and financially, and cause them severe, inhuman, excruciating pain. As the cancer slowly spreads, it eats them alive and they die a horrific death. For most Americans who have cancer... these fears quickly become their reality.

Today millions and millions of people are diagnosed with cancer every year. Over 1 million Americans last year were diagnosed with just skin cancer alone. Cancer is now the # 2 killer of Americans, but depending on whose statistics you read, cancer may actually be the # 1 killer. Around 1900, it was believed that about 1 out of 25 Americans got cancer in their lifetime. Today, every other adult American male will get cancer in his lifetime, and every third woman.

The truth is that most cancers are fairly modern diseases that have been created by modern living. Medical researchers estimate that over 80% of all cancers are caused by our unhealthy modern lifestyle. The vast majority of all cancers are caused by poisonous chemicals in our food, water, air and environment. Over 33% of all cancers are caused by an unhealthy diet and a lack of exercise alone. In my clinic I observed that in addition to these environmental causes, there were literally hundreds of negative emotional poisons that caused cancer too, from shame and blame to fear, guilt, depression, anger, and just plain old stress. On the other hand, when my patients with cancer STOPPED making themselves sick and STARTED living a healthy lifestyle, this is NOT what happened to them. And not just a few isolated cases, but hundreds and hundreds of my patients healed their cancers. And not just a few types of cancer, but every cancer that I have heard of.

This statement is a very dangerous one for me to make, especially in America. Making this statement has caused my clinic to be shut down and also caused my herbal products company, the American Botanical Pharmacy, to be closed on occasion. In case you are wondering about the protection offered by the 1st Amendment of the United States Constitution, guaranteeing us freedom of speech, this protection no longer applies to Dr. Schulze. And really no longer applies to any American who speaks the truth about cancer, especially about how it is created by the pollution, industrial waste and chemicals used by all of the top American corporations, let alone speaking about how easy it is to heal cancer, naturally, of course. But I'm not talking anymore. I'm going to let my patients and customers do the talking.

The very difficult job was to pick only a few people from the thousands of letters I receive, but I did, and I apologize to the many that I didn't print. So I picked out my patients or customers who were told by the medical doctors that they would be dead and that their cancer would kill them years ago. But instead they healed themselves naturally. Let these people be your teachers instead of me. They have great knowledge and experience to share, which they will do in chapter 10 of this book.

Chapter Ten

Patient & Customer Success Stories

Interview by Hilda Ganjian (an employee of Dr. Schulze's American Botanical Pharmacy)

Martin is a 62 year old male that resides in Jasper, FL and is retired from the airline industry. He was diagnosed in August 1997 with Waldenstrom's Macroglobulinemia, which is a rare malignant blood cell disease similar to Leukemia. He was predicted to die only a few months later, but 6 years later he is very alive and healthy.

"What symptoms did you have that told you something was wrong"

Oh, well, there were many at the time. Of course, I didn't realize they were symptoms. You don't realize them until you look back. One of them was, in my particular cancer, fatigue. High Blood Pressure. Oh, it just went on and on and on. Blacking out spells. Lost ability to think clearly. And that's all because my disease produces very thick blood, so your blood can't reach your smaller capillaries up in your brain and in your eyes and what have you. So all those symptoms and none of the doctors, of course, knew what it was.

"So what disease did the medical doctors diagnose you with?"

Macroglobulinemia

"What a long name."

Well, it's a very rare cancer. It affects only five out of one hundred thousand people. So I was lucky, I guess. But anyhow, it affects the bone marrow, so it's sort of like a bone marrow and blood cancer.

"Did you have more than one medical opinion?"

Yes. I went to two different doctors.

"What was the date of the diagnosis?"

It was around August of '97.

"What was their prognosis?"

Well, the prognosis with this disease is five years. But the bad news was, they said that I'd already had it for many years. So I was like on minus zero. I was out of time. Oh, another thing… another symptom was my blood had become so thick that it burst vessels in my kidneys, and I was urinating straight blood for about two months, and they didn't even know what the heck it was. So I really… I was out of time. I had no time left. I was dead.

"Did you receive any medical treatment?"

I was trying to listen to the doctors and so I started with the chemotherapy, because they told me that was the only way. I had chemotherapy three times.

"What was the outcome of this treatment?"

Well, the outcome was that my cancer was still there. The chemotherapy was ineffective against it. What was worse was now the chemotherapy had destroyed 80% of my bone marrow. I had only twenty percent of my bone marrow remaining, and they told me that it might not ever come back. And they said… the doctor told me at the time that I was getting very difficult to treat, as he put it. He said that if he gave me any more chemotherapy drugs that I would die, but then on the other hand, if he didn't I would probably die also. So with those odds I left his office and never came back.

"What year was the treatment?"

I got the chemo in 1997 through the first part of 1998.

"What did you do next?"

Well, I started putting together a hodgepodge health program of my own, just going from health food store to health food store, not knowing what the heck I was doing.

"Why did you decide to investigate Natural Healing?"

I was trying to put something together myself. I knew that the medical treatment was not working, in fact I was getting worse, and anyhow, at that time was when I discovered Dr. Schulze.

"How did you discover Dr. Schulze?"

Well, it was actually a mailer that Sam Biser had sent out that I had laying around for over a month, about a book called 'Curing with Cayenne' where he interviewed Dr. Schulze. So I read it and it was really interesting. So then I started seeing the light there and so I sent for Sam Biser's 'Save Your Life Video Collection' and went through all of that, and then I ordered all of Dr. Schulze's Herbal Incurables Programs.

"So out of Dr. Schulze's Natural Healing Programs and formulas, which ones did you use? Which programs did you do?"

At first, I was trying to be a little bit selective, and I realized in studying his material that that really wasn't the wise thing to do, so then I went back to square one and did everything that I was supposed to do.

"So you just kind of experimented with some SuperFood and maybe intestinal cleansing?"

Well, initially I went through huge amounts of garlic. And cayenne. And then SuperFood. But then I realized that I also had to do the intestinal # 1 and # 2, and do the Liver and Kidney detoxes and all that, and I've done those probably about… oh, I don't even know how many times I've done them. A lot. In fact, last month I just did another thirty-day Incurables Program, just for insurance.

"How long did you use the programs and the herbal formula?"

I'm still using them. I use all of his products. I just use them on an as needed basis now. But the cayenne and the SuperFood regularly. And of course the garlic. But I also take… when it's time to do the cleanse, I do the Liver/Gallbladder and the Kidney Detox and all that. And we drink a lot of his Detox Tea. In fact, I got some soaking right now.

"What were the results?"

Well, for somebody that wasn't supposed to be here, I feel pretty good. I'm thankful for every day, and I enjoy breathing. I do a lot of deep breathing and I do a lot of walking and exercise when I can. And I remember in '97 that I didn't think that I was going to be able to do that ever again.

"Have you had any relapses?"

Well, occasionally I feel like… I don't know if it's just that I'm paranoid or what, but occasionally I feel like I've got a symptom coming on or something, and that's when I just turn it up a little bit. Like last month I did the Incurables Program. If I feel like it might be one of my early, early symptoms that I had and didn't know what they were, I'll go ahead and turn it up. And the body knows what to do at that point.

"What would you like to say to our readers who are thinking about trying Natural Healing and Herbal Medicine?"

Well, I would have given anything at the time, when I was diagnosed and felt like a lost soul… my wife and I both did… to have had something like this to fall back on. Before I got exposed to chemotherapy. If I had known then what I know now, I would never have had a drop of chemotherapy put in me. And what I would say is, try this first. Because it does work. But you have to be a believer. If people are going to start second-guessing everything, their chances aren't as good.

You really have to have everything to gain by trying the natural healing method first. And then if for some reason if you're not satisfied, then you can always go see the other guys. But if I... I would have given anything, my wife and I, if we would have had this knowledge that we have now... back then. Because, to me, it works. It's just the way Dr. Schulze puts it. You stop doing what harmed you in the first place, and then start putting in some good stuff. And your body knows what to do with it. It'll heal itself. And a lot of loving thoughts.

"Do you have any words of advice for anyone who is already on Dr. Schulze's Incurables Program?"

This is a lifetime commitment. This is not a part-time job. If you value your health, then you know that it's a full-time job. And you need to be aware that you can't slide back to your old ways or you're going to get sick again. Your body's already proved that it can get sick. That would be my advice, make sure you stay on it.

And experiment with it a little bit. Learn your own... Don't be afraid to try a few things on your own. Dr. Schulze encourages that, too.

"Like the garlic."

That's a lot of garlic. Twenty or thirty cloves is really just an average. Some days I did more than that.

"How many would be your highest?"

I would probably say about forty. I probably did forty a few days. One thing I also did is I would maybe one day a week, like Sundays, and not take any, kind of a dry-out, because I feel like any herb is more effective if you lay off of it periodically. That's just my feeling, my inner voice talking to me there. But I just lay off, and then I go back to it really hard. But never more than a day or two. And I drink a lot of water. A lot of distilled water. And I got a Vita-Mixer going, and a Champion juicer going constantly. Even when I'm not feeling bad. That's just part of our life.

"Do you have any final comments or messages you would like to pass along to our readers?"

Well, I don't feel like I would have been here if it hadn't been for Dr. Schulze. I feel like I owe him my life. And I would support anything that he comes up with. Because I feel like he's the real deal. And we need a lot more people like him around.

"I couldn't agree with you more, because he saved me also."

He did?

"Yeah."

Oh, God bless you. Well, you know how I feel then.

"Very grateful. And honored to be on the same planet as Dr. Schulze."

Yeah, and, you know, when you listen to his story, isn't it a miracle that he's even here?

"Exactly. We are blessed."

He's doing what he's here for.

"Well, thank you. I really appreciate your time, and it seems like you've done all of the herbs and programs. That's beautiful."

I've tried just about everything, some of it harder than others. But I didn't do much skipping around. I started that at first, and then I realized that wasn't the way to go.

"As you said, it is a lifetime…"

Yeah. Like the hot and cold showers, I do them every day.

"That is so awesome."

And sometimes I'm really not in the mood for them, because I know the water. Like right now, tomorrow morning it's supposed to be twenty-nine degrees here. And I know my water is going to be about that temperature when I shower this afternoon.

"That's going to be really cold water."

It's going to be a good one. But I still do it.

"This is so great, because it's even motivating me to do some of this stuff that I have lacked. You know, sometimes you just feel like, I don't really need to do this. Like the hot and cold showers, and again, it's a part of your life right now."

That's it. You gotta just stay with it. By the way, how much do you have to pay Dr. Schulze to work for him?

"Isn't that the best question. I swear, I always say that if I could I would love to work for him for free. It's really, truly an honor, and every time I see Dr. Schulze I do tell him that, that it's really an honor to work for him."

I'm always telling my wife that I would like to pay Dr. Schulze to be his gardener. Just being his gardener and playing around in his fruits and vegetables all day.

Interviewed by Adam Loef, CEO of Dr. Schulze's American Botanical Pharmacy

---

Jim S., DDS is a 57 year old male from Fresno, CA and is a dentist. He was diagnosed in February 1995 with Non-Hodgkins Lympoma, which is a malignant cancer of the immune system, including lymph nodes, bone marrow, liver, spleen and the gastro-intestinal tract. He was predicted to die in the summer of 1995 after chemotherapy treatment failed and was only given a 20% chance to live if he did stem call treatment, which he declined. It is now eight and a half years later and he is living and healthy.

"What symptoms did you have that told you something was wrong?"

Kind of vague pain in my gut, almost like I had the flu which accelerated rapidly into pain that shot down from my shoulder into my gut to my liver, down around my abdomen. It actually felt like I was stabbed with a sword, although I hadn't been stabbed with a sword, but it felt like it.

"How long did you experience that pain before you sought advice?"

It was short, about a week because the pain was severe.

"Did the pain come on abruptly?"

Yes. I remember being in a drug store and telling my wife I am going to take this antacid medication. I said if the pain doesn't get better I am going to go to the doctor. The pain didn't get better and I went to the doctor. I went to a Gastroenterologist who then referred me to an Oncologist.

"What disease did the medical doctors diagnose you with?"

Non-Hodgkin's Lymphoma. Previously, in October 1994, I had a medical physical with blood tests and was given a clean bill of health. In February 1995 when the severe pain wouldn't go away I went to see my doctor. The first thing is they did a blood panel again and a panel and the numbers were way off from my physical three months earlier. So the doctors were really suspicious. They did the ultrasound and, probably inappropriately, the lady doing it felt she could share the outcome with me. You know they are not supposed to show the patient what is going on, but they did and she turned the monitor around and showed me all these tumors that were obvious. Shortly thereafter I had a CAT scan and the doctors discovered I had 5 tumors. I believe the largest was 6 inches by 5 inches by 5 inches. The tumors were in my liver and pancreas. This was around the first of February 1995. I was diagnosed with Non-Hodgkin's Lymphoma.

"What was their prognosis?"

My Oncologist recommended a 6 month program of chemotherapy with a 50/50 chance of survival.

"Did you receive any medical treatment?"

Well, every month the Oncologist told me I was doing great, but at the end of the 6th month his exact words were: "You failed conventional chemotherapy. You are going to die. The only thing we can do is a stem cell transplant and you'll only have a 20% chance of surviving, even with this treatment." (A stem cell transplant is where the medical doctors remove important immune cells from your body. They do this because the new, more powerful chemotherapy kills your immune system. Then after the chemotherapy hopefully kills all of the cancer and tumors, but not you, they can hopefully put your immune cells back into your blood.) This type of treatment has always seemed to me like two kids playing behind a garage with a cat or something. It seems so crude. I also believed that what you eat made a difference in your health. But when I started to do the chemo I asked my medical doctor what I should eat and he said it didn't matter. He said I could eat anything I wanted to. Actually, that was my first feeling that what this doctor was saying didn't make any sense to me.

"Why did you decide to choose Natural Healing and Herbal Medicine?"

I was trying to talk myself into this stem cell transplant even though it just didn't make sense, but I had nothing else going on at that time. But at the same time the chemo made me so sick, it depleted my immune system to the point where I couldn't walk without my wife helping me. I was like an 80-year-old and my life was looking pretty bleak to me. It was at that point that my wife said we need to try something else. It was her motivation.

I didn't want to do the stem cell therapy. I thought I was going to die. I knew and had heard how debilitating stem cell transplants were.

"How did you discover Dr. Schulze?"

I received a video from a friend about stem cell therapy and how debilitating it was. He wanted me to do Natural Healing. When my wife said we should try something else, we invited this friend in and that is when I got started on Natural Healing. I went pretty hog natural. I didn't eat any cooked food. I had carrot juice with a little bit of fresh apple juice several times per day. Then a friend said, "You want to do herbal cleansing," so I went to do a treatment program at a clinic up in Northern California and this is where I was introduced to Dr. Schulze's 5-Day Cleansing and Detoxification Programs.

"What did you do there?"

The woman who ran the clinic was a big Dr. Schulze follower. At this clinic they were talking about this black rubber that is going to come out of my bowel with the colon cleanse. But I thought I was clean after doing 4 months of colonics, coffee enemas, so at first I said that this stuff is not going to come out of me, I was clean. But I did a thorough herbal bowel cleansing anyway. I actually filtered my poop and the stuff I saw come out of my body made me a believer. Sure enough, when I filtered my poop I had it just like everyone else. That really made me a believer in herbal cleansing so then I did the liver cleansing next and when I filtered my poop, I found gallstones.

"What made you choose Dr. Schulze's program?"

The woman who ran the treatment facility in Northern California turned me onto Dr. Schulze. I started to play his tapes and I ate it up. As you know, in the Natural Healing world there's a plethora of information out there that is a little bit varied, not put together well. I liked Dr. Schulze because he had put it together.

"Which of Dr. Schulze's Natural Healing Programs or Herbal Formula did you use?"

SuperFood, Intestinal Formula # 1, Intestinal Formula # 2, Echinacea (I have taken Echinacea every day for probably 6 years), 5-Day Liver Detoxification and Cleansing Program and the Kidney Cleanse.

"What were the results?"

I just feel better and better.

"How long ago was that?"

Eight years ago.

"Have you had any relapses?"

No.

Dr. Schulze's note: What happened to Jim's 5 tumors? Jim sent a letter stating the details of his healing miracle: "I started to believe so much in natural healing and herbal medicine that I postponed my stem-cell transplant (which my oncologist was pressuring me to do before Christmas 1995!). We saw him in February 1996. Remarkably, without any chemotherapy since early December, my tumors were slightly smaller. This was great news! It blew the oncologist's mind. However, he didn't have an explanation but he had to admit that what we were doing was helping. Gradually, because of the friction of my opposing belief system, I decided not to return for further medical treatment. In November 1996 I had my last CAT scan. It showed that my tumors were very small. My oncologist stated, 'You don't have cancer anymore, because cancer grows! You're in remission!'"

"What would you like to say to any readers who are thinking about trying Natural Healing and Herbal Medicine?"

Since my healing I have talked to many other cancer patients, most receiving the same type of conventional chemotherapy treatment that I initially received, for all different types of cancer. Few have tried this nutritional approach, but those who have tried natural healing had very positive results! I want you to know that you, your loved ones, friends, and acquaintances don't have to choose the traumatic conventional oncology arsenal of chemotherapy (poisonous chemicals), radiation (Burning tissue), or surgery (often traumatic mutilation).

"Do you have any words of advice for anyone who is already on Dr. Schulze's Incurables Program?"

Do his Incurables Program with the same intensity you would like to live.

"Do you have any final comments or messages you would like to pass along to the readers?"

I think sometimes in life we have opportunities that are very unique and Dr. Schulze is one of them. It would be a shame not to take advantage of it and his products and programs. I think there is just the one thing about Dr. Schulze; it is that there is no one like him. If this guy went away there is no one to fill that void.

———

The following is a letter received from Toni L. who resides in Newport Beach, CA and is a Wild Animal Behaviorist and Writer. She was diagnosed in 1997 as having Breast Cancer and predicted to die only four and a half months later. It is now six years later and she is currently healthy and on a safari in East Africa working.

In 1997 I was diagnosed with breast cancer. The doctor told me I was a worst case scenario and would be dead in four-and-a half months without surgery.

My daughter worked at a breast cancer lab and was terrified for me by what she knew. Because of her fear, the fear of my friends, the steady drumbeat of the doctor and my own ignorance, I had the breast removed. Later I met with the Oncologist. He said, "I'm sorry to tell you, the final lab reports show your central lymph nodes are lit up!" (Editor's note: This means the cancer has metastasized and spread throughout her body.) "We are going to bomb you with chemo and radiation." I said, "No you are not!" Then I walked out. My medical doctor followed me down the hall, screaming, "If you don't do this, you'll die!"

My mother and sister died of breast cancer. Since I have a daughter and three granddaughters, I decided it was going to stop with me! I sent in search of those who healed themselves through alternative medicine. A friend told me about Dr. Schulze and gave me the number of the American Botanical Pharmacy.

Within a week I changed my life! I became a vegan-vegetarian, juiced 3 times a day, used SuperFood, Echinacea Plus, the Intestinal Cleansing Program, the Liver Flush and Kidney and Bladder Flush. I religiously watched the "Save Your Life" videos over and over again, drilling them into my head, preparing for the Incurables Program. At the end of the week I believed everything Dr. Schulze said.

In 1998 I had lab work done. Before the doctor read me the results, he asked about my diet. "Because I haven't seen blood as good as yours in years," he said.

I told him I was an organic, vegan-vegetarian who follows Dr. Richard Schulze's program. He said, "You break the records. You are healthy as a horse. Nothing bad could survive in your blood."

Six cancer-free years later, I am an Incurables testimonial. Thank you.

————

Interview by Hilda Ganjian (an employee of Dr. Schulze's American Botanical Pharmacy)

Brenda Michaels is a 54 your old female that resides in the Seattle, WA area and is a Speaker, Writer, Counselor, and Radio host. She has been diagnosed with Cervical cancer in 1975, cancer of the left breast in 1988, cancer of the right breast in 1989, and Lymph Node cancer in 1989 and predicted to die in 1990. It has been 14 years later and Brenda is currently extremely healthy and is the co-host of Conscious Talk, a radio show broadcasting Sundays 8-10pm on KKNW 1050AM in Seattle. (or go to to hear her.)

Editor's Note: Twenty-eight years ago, in 1975, Brenda was diagnosed with cancer of the uterus. The medical doctors did a hysterectomy and removed her uterus. Afterwards the doctors said she was fine.

"What symptoms did you have that told you something was wrong?"

The physical symptoms were fatigue and an extreme burning pain in my breast. I had some swelling there that eventually became a rather large lump that I could feel when I touched my breast. But it started out as a burning pain in that area.

"What disease did the medical doctors diagnose you with?"

The first time, they diagnosed me with an infection alongside of my nipple on the left breast. They said I had an infected milk gland, and they thought the burning was from the infection and they gave them antibiotics. And actually the antibiotics helped a little bit, which led them to continue to believe that's what it was. They even did a mammogram and an ultrasound. They continued to tell me that it was an infected milk gland.

"Did you have more than one medical opinion?"

I saw four different doctors in two years that gave me all a very similar diagnosis. And then finally, when I moved to L.A., and was doing a modeling job for a lady that I used to work for in Beverly Hills, she asked me what was wrong with me. She said that my sparkle was missing, and I told her it was my breast, and she got this really panicked, fearful look on her face and said, what do you mean, your breast? And I told her I had a lump in my breast, and she insisted on seeing the breast and touching the lump, and she just panicked and she got me in touch with a breast surgeon in Beverly Hills. And he was the first doctor that even suggested that I get a biopsy of the lump in my breast with a needle. He sent a runner with the needle biopsy to the lab, and he made me wait there to get the lab results back, because he was so sure that this lump was malignant. And I waited in his office for almost three hours. And when he came in, his whole body language… I knew what he was going to tell me. He said I had breast cancer.

"What was the date of diagnosis?"

October of 1988.

"What was the doctor's prognosis?"

All he told me was that until they could get in there surgically he didn't know what my chances were. And he said we need to schedule the surgery right away. And we did. I was in the hospital five days later and they removed my breast. They took the entire breast, including the whole nipple since it was infected.

"Did you receive any other medical treatment?"

They wanted to put me on chemotherapy, and I said no. And they wanted me to use Tamoxifin and I said I wasn't open to it. He sent me to two different oncologists. And I had a really bad experience with the first oncologist, who was just very insincere and very… he scolded me, and said that I was being prideful, that I didn't want to lose my hair, that I was more concerned about how I looked than the fact that my life was at stake. Which was not true. I did not feel like I wanted to do chemotherapy. I didn't know what else to do at the time, but I felt like I didn't want to do that. So the second oncologist he sent me to, I allowed to talk me into taking the Tamoxifin Chemotherapy.

"What was the outcome of your chemotherapy treatment?"

Well, I did not feel good on it. I took it for four months, and there was just something in me that just said this is not good for me. And I stopped taking it, and of course my oncologist was furious. But I said, I can't do this. I don't feel good, it doesn't feel right to be doing this. And he sort of scolded me a little bit. But he didn't argue too much with me because I was going in every so many months to get my blood tested, and have these tests done, and I had my lungs X-rayed and my bones scanned, and everything was clear, so he was telling me as far as he was concerned, since there wasn't lymph node involvement that this particular tumor was contained.

He thought I was going to be OK. But I kept telling him, like six or seven months down the road, I said, I'm still tired, I still don't feel right, and I don't understand why. And he kept telling me that I hadn't recovered from the surgery and chemotherapy. But I kept thinking, geez, I was working out every day, I was in good shape before I went into this, and I thought I should be feeling better than this. There was a little unsettling in me. I had this feeling that something was wrong, something was off. And of course in those days back then, I didn't listen to my feelings, instead I listened to the medical doctors. I kept insisting that I didn't feel good and he kept insisting that I would eventually

"What year was this treatment?"

This was 1989. In October of 1989, a year after I had my first surgery, my doctor scheduled me for a mammogram of my right breast. And when he took a mammogram of it and couldn't find anything at that time, and that was when I was losing my left breast, nobody said another word about it. Well, a year later when they did a mammogram they found little tiny specks under the scar, right beneath the scar. Little pinhead specks that looked suspicious to the radiologist. So the radiologist sent my report over to my oncologist and he called me up and said, I'm sorry to say this but we need to biopsy your right breast. And it was deep in the tissue, so I had to go into surgery again. And the biopsy confirmed malignant cancer in my right breast now and also in four lymph nodes. So I had surgery to remove my right breast, and they removed fifteen lymph nodes and there was cancer in four of them.

"What was your medical prognosis after the surgery?"

His prognosis was... my doctor was insisting that I do more chemotherapy, that I had no choice, and he told me that he felt if I would do the chemotherapy he could give me at least five years and maybe more. But he said that if I did not do the chemotherapy, he said that he couldn't even guarantee me a year before the cancer would metastasize and kill me.

"What year was the prognosis?"

Around 1989.

"Why did you decide to choose Natural Healing and Herbal Medicine?"

Everything in me, when I sat with chemotherapy, and even said that word to myself, every cell in my body… it's like I would find this fist in my gut, and every cell in my body would tense up. It was like I knew if I paid attention to what my body was saying, chemotherapy was not the answer for me. I was, for the first time, paying attention and listening to myself. And when I told my doctor that, he poo-pooed it like you could not believe. And scolded me, like the other guy had, and said that I was being silly and foolish and I was fooling around with my life. And I said, no, I really believed that if I did the chemotherapy I would lose my life. And that's how it felt to me. And he asked me what I was going to do, and at that point I didn't know. I said, I don't know, but I'm not going to follow this medical protocol.

And I walked out of his office, and he told me if I walked out that he could no longer be responsible for me, and it's the first time I realized that I needed to be responsible for me instead of giving him that power. And that's when I started to take charge of my healing process.

"How did you discover Dr. Schulze?"

I found out about Dr. Schulze about a year and a half later. It was probably 1992. Somebody told me about Dr. Schulze, and the way they spoke about him, there was an energy that left an impression on me, and a little voice in me said that I had to get in contact with him. So I did.

"And what made you choose Dr. Schulze's program?"

Dr. Schulze had his practice then so I called him personally, and I talked to him on the phone. Then, I went down and visited him. I ended up staying at his house for five days, doing herbs and doing some cleansing. He even took me for a walk on the beach and literally threw me in the ocean. Spending a few days with him made me a believer. I realized that I was on the right track. I was on the track to reclaiming my health and rebalancing my body and giving it the environment it needed in order to heal. But I also realized I needed to work on the emotional and spiritual roots of my disease as well. And I did that too.

"What of Dr. Schulze's Natural Healing Programs or Herbal Formula did you use?"

His Incurables Program. I did it partially because I was still doing Dr. Gonzalez's programs, so he gave me parts of it to do that I added to Dr. Gonzalez's program.

"So you did Dr. Schulze's Intestinal cleansing, Liver flush and cleanse?"

Oh, yeah.

"The hot and cold hydrotherapy?"

Yes. Taking herbs, all types of herbs. And eating organically. And eating vegetarian. And eating clean food. And doing the hot and cold showers. All of that.

"Juice-fasting?"

Oh, yes. Oh, tons of juicing. I still do tons of juicing. Well, it's a lifestyle. What you really realize when you begin to walk a healing path is that a healing path is really the natural path of life and that you're in the flow of life and that flow is being in harmony with nature and all of those elements instead of out of harmony. And it's a lifestyle.

"And how long did you use Dr. Schulze's programs and herbal formulae?"

At least a couple of years. And I still use his programs and herbal formula to this day. You know, me and my husband still do the cleanses four times a year. And we still use Dr. Schulze's herbs, and follow his 5-Day Cleansing and Detoxification Program for the liver and that type of thing. I still do his Intestinal Formula cleanse # 1, and when I do a heavy cleanse I use the # 2.

My husband has taken his Heart Formula for a very long time and didn't have to have an angioplasty. He developed heart disease, and he started taking Dr. Schulze's Heart Formula, and he moved past all of that. We do his cold and flu formulas... I mean, we do just about everything he's got.

"What were the results?"

Oh, god, I'm healthy. I'm very healthy. I'm the healthiest I've ever been. You know, Dr. Schulze is absolutely right when he says, in order to heal your body and your life all you have to do is stop doing what you're doing that makes you sick and make different choices. And that's the truth. But you have to be honest about what you're doing. And you have to be willing to let it go for something better.

And what stops people from healing themselves is the fear of letting go of those habitual patterns that they're in. Even as much as they want to be well, that fear overwhelms them and I believe it's an absolutely catatonic state for a lot of people. And I had such a passion to get well, and not just physically but emotionally and spiritually. It just became a passion for me as I began to live it. It just brought so much joy and inner peace to my life that waking it, living it... it was all just one in the same eventually.

So my cancer... the disease in and of itself was an incredible opportunity and gift in my life for a lot of growth. And it continues. It continues to be a gift. It connected me to Dr. Schulze, whom I dearly love as... not only as a doctor, but as a human being, one human soul to another. And it's introduced me to a whole different lifestyle that uplifts me, and a lifestyle that... I'm honest in my life, I walk with more integrity, I honor my body, I honor myself, I honor my feelings.

"Have you had any relapses?"

No.

"What would you like to say to the readers who are thinking about trying Natural Healing and Herbal Medicine?"

That it is the most powerful, empowering gift they can give to themselves. Nobody can give it to them. They have to give it to themselves.

"And that's where the responsibility comes in."

That's right. There is no wellness without self-responsibility. There is no wellness without integrity. There is no wellness without honorability, and that means honoring yourself first and honoring others and their path. Because all of that leads to a breakdown on an emotional and spiritual level that sets the body up for disease.

"A customer always tells me, the body is your temple, and you are the one that is going to take care of that temple."

That's right. Nobody does it for you. And we don't catch disease. We open up and... what we do is create the circumstances that allow disease to manifest. And we need to be responsible not from a place of guilt and shame but from a place of my god, look how powerful I am to do this. Now if I stop doing what created those circumstances and did this, look what I can create.

"Do you have any words of advice for anyone who is already on Dr. Schulze's Incurables Program?"

Absolutely, unequivocally, stick with it. Embrace it. Appreciate it. Thank God for it. Because it is the only way. It's the only way. The other ways are band-aids. Only band-aids. I don't believe in cures. I believe in healing. And the only healing that can happen is if you walk that path. And that's what you can share by demonstration with everybody else.

"Do you have any final comments or messages you would like to pass along to our readers?"

I just want to say that whatever challenges that they are facing, if they can see those challenges as the incredible opportunities and gifts that they truly are, and that this is what their soul invoked for them in this lifetime, to move through and grow through and be willing to shift and transform themselves through. This is their blessing. There is no greater walk on this planet. Dr. Schulze walks this, and it's one of the reasons I love him dearly and highly respect him, because he knows it, and he walks it.

———

The following is an email from DaveB that was posted on an internet Health Forum discussing Dr. Schultze's herbal products.

"I used to get 3 severe colds every winter. They always started the same way. I would get a dry, scratchy sore throat at night followed by nasal congestion the next day. I would get one in late November or early December, one in late January or early
February and one in March. This has been going on for over ten years.

Last winter, in early December, I came home from work one night about 10:30 pm. My throat was dry and sore but I thought it was due to the extremely dry air in the building I was in and all the talking I had done that night. I drank some water and went to bed thinking that I would be fine in the morning. I woke up about 2:30 am with a cough that wouldn't stop and I noticed my nose was getting stuffed. I got up and took two whole droppers full of Dr. Schulze's Echinacea Plus mixed with one whole dropper full of his SuperTonic in a Dixie cup of distilled water and went back to bed.

I woke up at my normal time of 6:30 am and felt even worse than I did at 2:30. My throat was so sore that I could barely swallow, my cough was non-stop and my nose was filled again. I decided it was time to get serious. The first thing I did was to take a whole dropper full of Dr. Schulze's Throat/Tonsil tonic and squirt it directly, full strength on the back of my tongue and swallow it. That provided almost instant relief for the sore throat. Then I took the juice from two whole lemons and two whole limes and mixed them with 24 ounces of distilled water and drank it all. Then I got in the shower and applied some hot/cold hydrotherapy, scalding hot to ice cold seven times. When I got out of the shower, I mixed eight whole droppers full of Echinacea Plus with four whole droppers full of SuperTonic and four whole droppers full of Dr. Schulze's Sinus/Lung tonic with some distilled water and drank it. About a half hour later I mixed 8 ounces of orange juice with 8 ounces of distilled water in a blender with a banana and two heaping tablespoons of SuperFood. Over the next few hours I drank a gallon of distilled water and urinated almost every twenty minutes. I also took the Echinacea Plus with SuperTonic a couple more times. By lunchtime, 12:00, my symptoms were gone completely and didn't return until February when I repeated the process with similar results."

Cold Sheet Treatment Success Stories:

A man with thyroid cancer decided to have his rapidly growing malignant tumor, which was wrapped around his thyroid, treated. Although his doctors wanted to operate, he finally chose the Cold Sheet Treatment instead. If the doctors did operate, they planned to not only remove his thyroid but also his larynx and he would never speak again. His tumor was so large that they planned to remove a large part of his throat. He told them he wanted to think it over, and they said he would be dead in days if he didn't get the operation right away.

His neck tumor was about two inches wide when he took the cold sheet treatment. The first morning after his first Cold Sheet Treatment the tumor had shrunk 50% to only one inch. By the end of the week, his tumor was totally gone.

Dr. Schulze decided to do some deep body work on his throat during the last five minutes of the Cold Sheet Treatment while the patient was screaming. Before the last five minutes of treatment was up, the patient vomited up part of his tumor.

A young lady who was suffering from A. Lateral Sclerosis (Lou Gehrig's Disease) and Parkinson's Disease decided to get the Cold Sheet Treatment from Dr. Schultze. She suffered with muscle weakness, tremors and was degenerating rapidly. During her treatment, every muscle in her body went into a spasm and this was very painful for her, but the Lobelia Tincture she received eased her spasms and pain immediately. The next morning she had few signs of any neurological disorders and by the end of the week had no such signs at all. She was completely healed and two months later her original doctors were amazed.

Chapter Eleven

To Your Good Health

You've probably made a toast to someone's good health while drinking wine or other type of beverage. We say, "Here's to your good health" and lift our glasses or touch glasses and then take a drink.

Unfortunately, most of us today don't really do what is necessary to have excellent health. We eat dead foods, drink alcoholic beverages, drink regular tea, eat dairy products, eggs, meat, and most of us are constipated, and our systems are clogged with old feces as well as new, and we consume sugar, candy, and numerous amounts of toxins and poisons, etc. The list goes on and on. We get sick and our doctors prescribe one or more drugs, and most of us probably do not realize that drugs are poisons and poisons always poison us and do not make us well. I recently read where a medical doctor offered a large reward to any doctor or anyone else who could prove that any drug would actually cure a disease. So far, there have been no takers.

I have no ax to grind against doctors. I believe they are necessary and that we have many really good doctors. I just believe that if they stick to the format of cut, burn, and poison, they may do more harm than good, but some doctors do use other methods of treatment. We certainly do need doctors to examine us, to diagnose our diseases, and tell us what ailments we have. We need them when we have been injured and sometimes to operate to correct a defect in our bodies.

For many years I have been a member of The National Health Federation. Our organization is in business to protect our rights to freedom of choice, to give us the right to choose our methods of treatment or to take no treatment at all. After I had been a member of the NHF a few years, and attended several of their conventions in Pasadena, CA, I was asked by a speaker if I would fill in for him since he had to leave for a while. I was glad to do so, and many of those in attendance told him that I did great, and pretty soon I was filling in for speakers who, for some reason or another, were unable to speak. Then I became a regular speaker and chose my subject, "Cancer Prevention and Cure." I spoke in Orlando, FL, Chicago, IL, San Francisco, CA and every year in Pasadena, CA. The National Health Federation is a wonderful organization with some of the most wonderful people in the world, but after speaking for 10 years, I decided to discontinue speaking for them. If you would like to know more about The National Health Federation, you may telephone them at 626-357-2181 or write them at: P.O. Box 688, Dept. 7, Monrovia, CA 91017.

I hardly ever go to see a medical doctor for any medical attention, but I do go sometimes. I have used two doctors for many years and believe that both of them were excellent and honest doctors. One of my doctors was named Leon Carter, Jr. and he just died during the last of June, of 2001 at age 71. My other doctor is named Jim and he is still very much alive. I believe that you should learn as much as possible and take care of yourself as well as you can, without the help of a medical doctor, if possible. I think you will be healthier if you do this, so I recommend that you learn to be self-sufficient as much as possible, and you will see why by what follows.

You've probably read in your newspaper that President Nixon and others have declared "war on cancer" but haven't you noticed that a higher and higher percentage of our people die of cancer each year? I consider the "war on cancer" to be a phony war because nothing ever happened to make me believe that a war was really being waged. All of the cancer news was bad. Let's look at some of the facts:

1. CHEMOTHERAPY AND LUNG CANCER

Adding chemotherapy to radiation therapy does not prolong survival in operable, non-small cell lung cancer, according to a large, randomized study published in the October 26 issue of the New England Journal of Medicine.

Two hundred and forty two patients were randomized to receive radiation therapy alone while 246 received radiation therapy plus chemotherapy. The median survival time was 39 months in the group given radiotherapy and 37 months in the group given both radiotherapy and chemotherapy. In other words, adding chemotherapy made the results slightly worse.

The authors, from the Eastern Cooperative Oncology Group, concluded that compared with radiotherapy alone, radiotherapy and chemotherapy does not prolong survival in lung cancer patients.

A major study was published in the Lancet, a British publication, in 1998, which analyzed the results in 2128 patients who received surgery plus radiation compared to surgery alone. The study indicated a 21% increase in risk of death of patients receiving radiation therapy. Harm was greatest among those who had early stage I or II lung cancer. This would seem to indicate that radiation therapy after the operation should be avoided. Surprisingly, some doctors who have read this information still choose to give radiation after the operation. Don't you think that the doctor should make this information available to the patient and let the patient decide if he or she wants to buck these statistics? If the doctor knows of these statistics, don't you think that if he goes ahead and operates without allowing the patient to decide which treatment to have, that this is absolutely dishonest?

2. FOOD MAY CURE YOUR CANCER

Here is a great idea you may start using right away. This message comes from a biochemist, name unknown.

Asparagus For Cancer. Several years ago, I learned of the discovery of Richard R. Vensel, D.D.S., that asparagus might cure cancer. Since then, I have worked with him on this project, and we have accumulated a number of favorable case histories. Here are a few examples.

Case No. 1. One man had an almost hopeless case of Hodgkins Disease (cancer of the lymph glands), and he was completely incapacitated. Within 1 year after starting the asparagus therapy, his doctors were unable to detect any signs of cancer, and he is back on a schedule of strenuous activities. (NOTE: His only treatment was with asparagus!)

Case No. 2 is a successful businessman now 68 years old, who suffered from cancer of the bladder for 16 years. After years of medical treatments, including cobalt (radiation) without improvement, he went on asparagus. Within 3 months, hospital examinations revealed that his bladder tumor had disappeared and that his kidneys were normal. Today he is at least as healthy as before the disease started.

Case No. 3 is a man who had lung cancer. On March 5, 1971, he was put on the operating table, where they found lung cancer so widely spread that it was inoperable. (Note by author: This sounds like it had metastasized.) The surgeons sewed him up and declared his case hopeless. On April 5, he heard about the asparagus therapy and immediately started taking it. By August, x-ray pictures revealed that all signs of the cancer had disappeared. He is back at his regular business routine.

Case No. 4 is a woman who was troubled for a number of years with skin cancer. She finally developed 7 different skin cancers which were diagnosed by a skin specialist as "advanced." Within 3 months after starting on asparagus, her skin specialist said that her skin looks fine- no more lesions.

This woman reports that the asparagus therapy also cured her kidney disease, which started in 1949. She had over 30 operations for kidney stones and was receiving government disability payments for "a terminal kidney condition- inoperable." She attributes the cure of this kidney trouble entirely to the asparagus therapy.

I was not surprised at this result, as a book "The Elements of Materia Medica" edited in 1854 by a professor at the University of Pennsylvania, states that asparagus was used as a popular remedy for kidney stones. He even refers to experiments made in 1739 on the power of asparagus to dissolve urinary stones.

We would have other case histories, but the Medical Establishment has interfered with our obtaining some of the records. I am, therefore, appealing to readers to spread the good news and help us to gather a large number of case histories that will overwhelm the medical skepticism about this unbelievably simple and natural remedy.

HOW TO USE ASPARAGUS

Asparagus should be cooked before using, and therefore canned asparagus is just as good as fresh. I have corresponded with the two leading canners of asparagus, Green Giant and Stokely, and I am satisfied that these brands contain no pesticides or preservatives. However, they do contain salt and water.

The cheapest form is the "cut spears." Open the can and dump into a blender. Liquefy at high speed to make a puree, and store in a refrigerator.

Give the patient 4 full tablespoons twice daily, morning and evening. (Patients usually show improvement in from 2 to 4 weeks.) It can be diluted with water and used as a cold or hot drink.

The suggested dosage is based on present experience, but certainly larger amounts can do no harm, and may be needed in some cases.

As a biochemist, I am convinced of the old saying, "what cures can prevent." Based on that theory, my wife and I have been using asparagus puree as a beverage with our meals. We take 2 tablespoons of the puree (diluted with water to suit our taste) with breakfast and with dinner. I take mine hot; my wife prefers hers cold.

For years we have made it a practice to have blood surveys taken as part of our regular check-ups. The last blood survey taken by a medical doctor who specializes in the nutritional approach to health, showed substantial improvements in all categories over the last one, and we can attribute the improvements to nothing but the asparagus drink.

Asparagus contains a good supply of proteins called "histones" which are believed to be active in controlling cell growth. For that reason, I believe asparagus can be said to contain a substance that I call "Cell Growth Normalizer." That accounts for its action on cancer and in acting as a general body tonic.

In any event, regardless of theory, asparagus used as we suggest, is a harmless substance. The FDA cannot prevent you from using it, and it may do much good.

As a biochemist, I have made an extensive study of all aspects of cancer, and all of the proposed cures. As a result, I am convinced that asparagus fits in better with the latest theories about cancer.

Note by author: Please send me any information you have if you have been cured of any disease by using asparagus. Send this information to the publisher of this book.

Note: The above information comes from a wonderful publication called "God's Physician's," a monthly publication which you may order for $25 per year from Rev. Tom Kopco at 149 North Dr., Dept. 7, Lake Wales, FL 33859, or by telephone 863-675-1489.

3. FISH OIL

Dr. Artemis Simopoulos, a medical doctor indicates that there have been numerous studies which indicate that fish oil decreases the size of animal tumors, the number of tumors and also diminished their ability to spread. In human beings, fish oil also suppressed pre-cancerous colon polyps. As a matter of fact, tests have indicated that in just two weeks of consumption of fish oil, signs of colon cancer were suppressed. Signs of colon cancer diminished in over 60% of the people tested. This seems to indicate that if we just use fish oil for our cancer every day, we can get it under control pretty fast. Of course, if you have cancer, there is no reason why we can't use more than one method of treatment.

We know that fish is loaded with vitamin D, so we take 5000 i.u. of vitamin D each day to supplement the fish oil. Both fish oil and vitamin D are good at preventing cancer as well as making it go away. It is surprising that the recommended daily amount to be taken is only 200 i.u., when the Japanese women take 1,200 i.u. per day. When they move to the U.S., their intake of vitamin D diminishes and many of them come down with cancer. Deaths among men who eat lots of fish are much lower if they eat fish regularly.

I like the fish oil as well as fish and flaxseed oil for keeping cancer away as well as to get rid of it. All of these are so beneficial in so many ways that we should all take them and never stop. As an example, if your HDL, the good cholesterol, is subnormal, you may boost it tremendously if you start eating fish rich in omega 3. You may also eat salmon, tuna, sardines, mackerel, and herring, to raise your HDL cholesterol. We not only raise our HDL but we lower our LDL, the bad cholesterol, as well as triglycerides by consuming omega 3 products.

I buy myself fish oil concentrate, which has Omega 3, produced by NOW and I get the 1,000 mg size softgels. This is very inexpensive, so I purchase the bottle with 200 softgels and the cost is only $8.95 plus sales taxes. (CAUTION: There is such a thing as too much of a good thing. I may take 5,000 i.u. of fish oil a day and only 1,000 i.u. of vitamin D that same day and the next day only take 3,000 i.u. of fish oil and 3,000 of vitamin D. Just don't overdo it.) Size 1,000 i.u. softgels of vitamin D, sold by Solgar, is recommended.

RHEUMATOID ARTHRITIS

If you are hampered with arthritis, you may just benefit in more ways than you can imagine by consuming fish oil, and other seafood products already named. When you consume fish oil, this has the effect of significantly reducing leukotriene B4, which is an inflammatory substance responsible for your arthritis symptoms. The daily dose needed is 3,000 to 5,000 mg of fish oil soft gels. Although most of the fish oils you will see in the vitamin store are only 300 mg, you already know you can purchase the 1,000 mg size NOW brand. After you have taken up to 5,000 mg of fish oil for only a short while, you should notice that your pain has tremendously diminished and you have regained much of your strength. An added benefit is that this may also suppress up to 55% of the chemicals called cytokines, which damage or destroy joints.

One man stated that he took numerous medicines prescribed by his doctor for the pain, and then he started eating three cans of sardines each week and this enabled him to eliminate the arthritis pain for over 10 years.

Some people find that taking only one 1,000 mg soft gel controls their pain, and others find that 2,000 mg or even more is needed. You may have to try several weeks of different amounts. If you also eat fish or other seafood, you may find you need less of the fish oil.

MIGRAINES

If you regularly consume fish, tuna, salmon, sardines, mackerel, or fish oil, you may eliminate your headaches. The last thing in the world you should take for a headache is aspirin. Dr. Bill Douglas once said, "If you are suffering with a headache caused by an aspirin deficiency, then you should take aspirin for it."

People who regularly suffer with migraines may prevent all future headaches by taking fish oil, and other seafood named. Tests have shown that it is effective in preventing headaches in at least 60 percent of the cases, but it greatly relieves them in the other cases. (Note: It will also help if you keep your colon clean.)

LUPUS

People with lupus found that this would also help them. One doctor advises them to eat sardines packed in sardine oil 3 times per week, but I would suggest that if this doesn't completely relieve them, they should experiment starting with 7 times a week and gradually reducing it to the point where they get help eating sardines less than 7 times per week.

OTHER AILMENTS HELPED BY FISH OIL

Here are some other instances where this seafood may help.

- Psoriasis
- Multiple Sclerosis
- Heart Attack- reduces by 50% your chances of dying from a heart attack. If you have already had a heart attack, this may reduce your chances of having another one.
- May prevent blood clots and stroke
- High Blood Pressure
- Colitis- I developed colitis and decided I didn't want the doctor to treat it, so I went and got 16 colonic irrigations, and this completely eliminated the problem.
- Crohn's Disease- fish oil helped Italian doctors to keep Crohn's Disease patients from having a relapse. (Note: colonic irrigations may halp alleviate Crohn's Disease)
- Raynaud's Disease
- Scleroderma
- Aging- may slow down the aging process

PREVENTING CANCER

Another way to prevent cancer is to take vitamin A every day. I recommend 5,000 i.u. per day of this vitamin and 10,000 i.u. per day of beta carotene, plus 5,000 i.u. of vitamin D.. If you take only 2,500 i.u. per day, you may still get cancer. I've never heard of anyone dying because he took an overdose of vitamins, have you. If I were dying of cancer, I would not hesitate to take 25,000 i.u. of vitamin A for a couple of weeks. I would also take 5000 i.u. of fish oil per day and 5000 i.u. of vitamin D for two weeks. Then I would reduce the amounts of each one to a reasonable level.

CHERRIES

Cherries are loaded with perillyl alcohol which blocks the formation of numerous cancers, including cancer of the skin, lungs, stomach, breasts and liver. They also contain quercetin, which is ranked as one of the most potent anti-cancer agents ever discovered. It has a tendency to cut off the enzymes that tumors and cancers need to grow. I recommend that you buy and take Quercetin capsules daily.

HIGH BLOOD PRESSURE

One way to bring down high blood pressure is to eat celery. Within a week, blood pressure dropped about 15% because eating celery does the trick. (Note: Take a 500 mg of calcium and 250 mg magnesium capsule shortly before bedtime. This will help reduce your blood pressure if it is high, and is also good for your heart.)

FAVA BEANS

One of the best foods you can ever eat if you have Parkinson's disease is fava beans according to "The Doctor's Book of Foods That Heal."

FLU SHOTS MAY BE DANGEROUS
Here are some remarks written by Dr. Richard Schulze:

"Last year pharmaceutical companies made about 85 million doses of the flu shot. This is big business. Do the math. We're talking BILLINS and BILLIONS of dollars. This year, there was lower than anticipated production yields of the vaccine and also a delay in getting it to the public. Thank God! Although some doctors and patients who can't get the vaccine might turn to general anti-viral drugs, the Center for Disease Control warns that this is an untested and expensive strategy ard could result in large numbers of people getting ill.

There are hundreds of known influenza viruses, over 200 common ones. They never come alone and each year sees a mixture of many old viruses along with some new mutated ones. Two years ago in America we saw the A/Sidney/05/97 virus along with the A/Bejing/262/95, the A/New Caledonia/20/99, the A/Bayern/07/95, then B/Bejing/184/93, the B/Yamanashi/166/98, the A/Moscow/10/00, the A/Panama/2007/00, A/Johannesburg/82/96 and a host of others. Last years vaccine cocktail was a blend of the A/New Caledonia/20/99, the A/Panama/2007/99 and the B/Yamanashi/166/98. And this year's toxic chemical blend flu shot contains A/Moscow/10/99 (H3N2), the B/Victoria/504/2000, the A/New Caldonia/20/99 (H1N1), the A/Panama/2007/99 (H3N2), B/Johannesburg/05/99, B/Guangdong/120/2000, and the B/Sichuan/379/99.

Medical doctors literally guess at which viruses they think might come around each year because the vaccines have to be prepared up to a year in advance. Even if they were exactly right with their guess of which virus blend to put in the shot, and even got the right proportions, that still doesn't account for the new kids on the block. Influenza vaccine history shows that often even if they guessed right, the virus mutates during the year rendering the "flu shot" impotent and you still get the new mutated virus.

INJECTING BLENDS OF VIRUSES INTO YOUR BODY CAN BE VERY DANGEROUS. I remember the swine flu vaccine. It made people sicker than the swine flu itself and left others dead. This was because influenza vaccines can cause Guillain-Barre Syndrome, the immediate inflammatory destruction of the nerve sheath which causes rapid paralysis that paralyzed many who got the swine flu vaccine. ALL VACCINES CAN ALSO CAUSE LIFE THREATENNG AND LETHAL ALLERGIC REACTIONS. The only safe and effective defense to influenza is having a strong offense, a strong immune system that can kill and make antibodies for any virus that ever existed and any new one that mutates. The key to a strong immune system is a healthy lifestyle. It also doesn't hurt to have some potent herbal tonics around, like Echinacea and Garlic, that will knock the socks off any virus.

Note by author: Dr. Bill Douglas claims that there are over 1,000 different kinds of flu which we may have to worry about, and there is no way anyone can tell which type it will be, so I recommend avoiding flu shots.

Chapter Twelve

Some Good Ideas

1. APPLE CIDAR VINEGAR (ACV) (Note: Buy organic, if possible)

MEMORY IMPROVEMENT

ACV is great for you because it has so many benefits. If you are over age 40, you might want to start taking it to improve your memory. As we age, we often find that our memories have become less and less perfect. I suggest that you take a glass of water with your meals with one teaspoonful of ACV therein. You might even want to take 2 spoonfuls in a glass of water sometimes, for your memory.

ASTHMA

If you have asthma, you may want to take one teaspoonful in a half glass of water and just sip it slowly for about one half hour each day. This may help especially if you improve your diet.

HEMOPHILIA

If you suffer from hemophilia (inability to clot blood) you may benefit by taking ACV with your meals. One teaspoonful in a glass of water with your meals should help your blood to start clotting, when necessary.

LOSING WEIGHT

If you are obese, you may want to lose weight. Try drinking a glass of water with each meal with one teaspoonful of ACV in each glass. If you also eat a handful of walnuts before your main meal each day in addition to taking ACV with the meal, it may help even more.

RETARDING OLD AGE

Taking ACV with your meals may help you in numerous ways. It may even help you to slow down the aging process.

HEARTBURN AND BELCHING

If you take ACV with your meals, it may even help overcome heartburn and belching.

FREQUENT URINATION

Try 2 teaspoonfuls with your meals until you get the urination under control. It may help to give you better control so that you don't have to get up during the night to urinate.

SORE THROAT

If you should develop sore throat, try gargling with a mouthful every hour and then spit out the gargle. Then take a swallow of the water with a spoonful of ACV in it. Do this every hour until it is consumed.

PROMOTES DIGESTION

Another benefit of taking water with ACV in it is it promotes digestion. It may help to make your blood of the right consistency.

PREVENTS PUTREFACTION

It may help you to avoid intestinal putrefaction.

REDUCES OVEREATING

It will actually help to curb your appetite and may help to reduce stenographer's seat. It may help you to lose weight where you most need to lose it.

LARYNGITIS

To reduce laryngitis, put 2 teaspoonfuls of ACV in a glass of water and do as suggested with sore throat except do this every half-hour for eight hours, or until you have noticed great improvement before the eight hours is up. Make more than 1 glass of water with ACV, if necessary.

FREQUENT NOSE BLEEDER

Of course, it may help frequent nose bleeders also. Drink it with your meals and see if it doesn't help you to avoid frequent nose bleeding.

2. GARLIC

In Numbers 11:5, the Lord mentions GARLIC, and he mentions many other foods which are great, if not the greatest, food He gives us for healing ourselves.

Among the many diseases it can protect us from is the bubonic plague, which was one of the all time worst diseases. When it hit a city, quite often everyone in the city died from it. This disease is so horrible that anyone who breathes the air into which others with the disease have been coughing can catch the disease. It sometimes only takes three days for them to die just from breathing the dangerous, polluted air.

There is the story about the four thieves in Marseilles, France in 1722, who entered the city and plundered and robbed the dying of money, jewels and valuables, and seemed unconcerned about the bubonic plague, which was so devastating. When the authorities waited on one side of the city to arrest them, they would leave from the other side. Finally, they were caught, convicted and sentenced to death, but the authorities offered to reduce their sentences if they would tell their secret as to how they survived during the plague. They explained they had soaked 50 cloves of garlic in some strong wine vinegar and rubbed this on their hands, arms, faces, and other body parts, drank some and even gargled with it. They probably swallowed some garlic also, and said that the plague left them alone. This information was posted by the Marseilles police in Marseilles and this enabled the survivors to resist the disease.

It may also help with some of the following problems: Epileptic seizures, consumption (now known as tuberculosis), asthma (mix garlic and hyssop together and blend into a tea), leprosy, gangrene, gonorrhea, bronchitis, lung abscesses, allergies, emphysema, staphylococci germs, dysentery, salmonella poisoning, cancer, brain infection, diabetes, liver problems, cystitis, constipation, diarrhea, earache, and others. It may help prevent clogged arteries, and reduce high blood pressure.

For a great book listing treatments for garlic problems, and many others, I recommend "Miracle Food Cures From the Bible" by Reese Dubin.

3. FLAX SEED OIL + LOW FAT COTTAGE CHEESE

Many decades before Dr. Johanna Budwig of Germany began her research, a number of scientists were already beginning to see a connection between good health and consuming an oil plus a protein combination. In the early 1900s, three people studied this problem to find the answer, but to no avail.

Otto Fritz Myerhoff discovered that linoleic fatty acids and sulphur rich proteins work perfectly together to help fatigued muscles recover from exercise and exertion. Unfortunately, he did not realize the significance of his discovery since linoleic acid was not known to be essential.

Otto H. Warburg, who was also a German, realized that a fatty substance was necessary to restart oxidation when it was low, as it is in cancer and diabetes. He tested a number of fatty acids but failed to test using linoleic acid, although he was familiar with it. He gave up when he did not get the results he expected.

Albert Von Szent-Gyorgi, of Hungary, discovered that sulphur rich proteins, when paired with linoleic acid take up oxygen, but he lacked the biochemical techniques to prove the identity of the components.

All three of these researchers were Nobel Prize winners, but missed the solution they were so close to because of insurmountable technical difficulties.

Dr. Budwig conducted numerous and time consuming tests to develop new techniques in dealing with the oil-protein question. She found that neither the essential fatty acids nor the sulphur proteins do the job alone. They only work if consumed together in the right ratios. They also need chromium.

She put her knowledge into practice and started treating diseased human patients, supplementing their diets with 2 tablespoons of cold pressed flaxseed oil combined with skim milk. She later substituted one quarter cup of quark (low fat cottage cheese) because of the higher incidence of sulphurated proteins and also because this is more palatable. With this treatment, she found that the yellowish-green substance in the patient's blood was replaced with a healthy red pigment, hemoglobin. The phosphatides returned and the lipoproteins reappeared. This caused the tumors to recede and eventually disappear;

anemia was alleviated, vital energy increased, and the patient recuperated. It took about 3 months for all of this to happen, but during this time, all symptoms of cancer, diabetes, and liver disease disappeared.

Information about Dr. Budwig came from "The Healthy Cell News" and you may contact them at 1-800-624-7114 to place an order for BIOSAN VITA FLAX, which has all the ingredients mentioned in above, i.e. FlaxSeed Oil, and cottage cheese or other sulphurated proteins. They are known as Nature's Distributors, 16508 EA. Laser Drive, Bldg. B, Dept. 7, Fountain Hills, AZ 85268.

One of my clients tried this for his diabetes, which had progressed so far that he had lost several toes due to gangrene, and his diabetes was cured. He still takes this so that it may never return.

4. ALZHEIMER'S DISEASE

We've all heard of Alzheimer's Disease and would like to think that no one in our family circle will ever develop it. Since we know that the authorities that are supposedly in the know believe that aluminum may be the one thing that triggers Alzheimer's Disease, we must make certain that we don't contribute to our own accumulation of aluminum in our systems and actually cause ourselves to get Alzheimer's Disease.

Of course, the first thing we must do is check our own pots and pans and throw out all of them which are made of aluminum. This is then a good start, but we must do more. The second thing you should do is make absolutely certain that you NEVER, NEVER, drink any soda pop from a can. If you do drink from an aluminum can, it is entirely possible that you will deposit 4 milligrams of aluminum inside your body each time you drink and this is well above the maximum safe limit. If you must drink soda pop, make certain you buy it in bottles or something other than cans. Alzheimer's is a terrible disease which will shorten your life and make you eventually entirely dependent on someone else. Your mind will diminish and you may some day not recognize your closest relatives. You literally lose your mind.

5. GOUT (A form of arthritis)

If you have gout, you may eventually develop excruciating pain in your big toe and find that one day you will be confined in a wheelchair. This is what happened to one man and he heard of a diet which consisted of eating at least 6 cherries (or more) each day for his gout. It was not long before he was up and walking. Numerous others who have tried this treatment agreed that it worked.

Suggestion: If you have access to fresh cherries, I would recommend that you buy them in preference to bottled cherries. Always go natural if you have a choice. Anytime that you can buy and eat some fruit the way the Lord made it, it is certainly better than buying processed fruit. You'll get better results as well.

6. CARROTS

When you eat carrots, sweet potatoes, pumpkins, and red peppers, you get beta-carotene. All of these are good for you. Beta-carotene is good against stroke, heart disease, cancer, and other diseases.

In one study, it was determined that just eating one carrot per day would cut your chances of getting a stroke by a whopping 68%. If you want beta carotene's protection against killer diseases, you will not get it from beta carotene supplements which you may buy in a health food store, but you will only get it by eating the carrot (or other foods rich in beta carotene) itself. Scientists claim that the reason for this is that carrots have over 500 siblings, which are known as carotenoids. So remember, if you take the vitamin pill, you sacrifice most of the benefits, but if you eat the carrot itself, you tremendously decrease your chances of having a stroke and you may even enjoy the taste of carrots. Fresh carrot juice may also be equally great for you. (Suggestion: If you want to eat carrots, be certain to buy organic carrots.)

7. HEADACHES

Dr. Richard Schulze writes a monthly newsletter, which is quite interesting. He covers many health subjects, and always does a magnificent job. Let's read what he says about headaches. "I had a patient come to me with severe migraines. They were so bad that she would even go blind during some of the attacks. Her daughter told me that sometimes she would fall to her knees in public, screaming that she couldn't take it anymore, or even blackout or faint. She went to her medical doctor who gave her some painkillers and the migraines went away, but eventually they came back. She asked the doctor for something stronger, he eventually prescribed narcotics. The pain went away, but eventually came back.

She then went to see an Oriental Medical Doctor who did acupuncture on her, stuck hundreds of needles in her, she said she felt like a human pincushion. The pain disappeared, but returned.

Out of frustration, she went to a friend's Chiropractic Doctor who noticed that her cervical vertebrae were subluxated. After a series of adjustments, her pain went away, but eventually it came back. Out of desperation, she went to a Rolfer, a great system of deep tissue body work, and he did some real restructuring of her neck muscles and tissue, in fact her whole body, and the pain was totally gone, but eventually it came back.

Finally she ended up at an herbalist. He prescribed her a classic old herbal formula for pain, actually a great effective formula and one that I used often in my clinic also. It was a miracle, her pain completely disappeared. GONE!.. but it eventually came back.

After 3 years of blinding pain, and seeing 16 different doctors and spending thousands of dollars on everything from electrode stimulators and biofeedback devices to drugs, herbs, vitamins, enzymes, colloidal silver and noni fruit drink, she finally crawled up to the doorstep of my clinic and told me her story.

Within the first 2 minutes of her very first visit, I asked her one of my favorite questions, how often do you have a bowel movement? It turned out she only went once or twice a week. I suggested that before we do anything, we do a thorough bowel cleansing routine for a couple of weeks. She was furious, she screamed at me and demanded I give her my migraine formula. She was literally sobbing, in tears, begging, pleading for relief. I gave her my Bowel Detoxification Program and sent her home.

After a few days she called me and told me that her migraines were gone right after an amazing pooping experience on the toilet, but was afraid they would return like they had done with ALL the other doctors and practitioners. Over the next few months, I put her through all of my programs and cleaned her colon out a few more times and the migraines have never returned. That was thirteen years ago. The problem with all of the doctors that she saw was that they were all focused on the pain in her head, about 3 feet above the real problem.

8. PAIN IN LUMBAR VERTEBRAE, SACRUM AND SCIATIC NERVE

Dr. Richard Schulze continues:

I had a lady come in to see me; she had been out of work, literally, flat on her back in pain for 2.5 years. She had pain in the lumbar vertebrae, sacrum, and sciatic nerve, EVERY DAY, ALL DAY. No work, not even housework, not even going shopping for a few groceries, she was 100% crippled, a total wreck. The medical doctors wanted to fuse her spine, maybe cut the sciatic nerves to relieve the pain.

This is a total dead end. She had many visits to her Chiropractor, along with Hatha Yoga, which are two of the best therapies for any spinal problem, and especially lower back problems, but got little results. The Osteopaths or Orthopedic treatments didn't help either, and she was at her wit's end. She even told me that she was contemplating killing herself.

Guess what? She was constipated! I put her on the bowel cleansing program and in less than a week all of her pain was gone, and never returned. She was shocked in disbelief. And she was really, really mad at all the doctors for overlooking something so simple, constipation. Her blocked, engorged, swollen colon was pressing on all the nerves in her lower back.

So even if a person thinks that their particular problem is unrelated to the colon, they might be wrong. A swollen, constipated, irritated bowel puts pressure on and infects everything around it. The nerves from the spine, run right next to the bowel before they go down the legs. I have had hundreds of patients with chronic back pain, sciatica, leg pain, and it all disappeared after a good bowel cleansing program.

No matter how far removed the problem seems from the colon, no matter how ridiculous it may seem to do a bowel cleansing program instead of brain surgery, cleanse the bowel first and see what happens.

Note by author: A young lady in my church was suffering with severe headaches. She is only a teenager, and I kept reading month after month that she was suffering with very severe headaches. I don't remember how long this had been going on but I believe it was more than a year. Finally, after I read it the next time, I decided that it was time that I do something about it. I saw her in church and told her that I wanted to talk with her, and asked her to get her mother to join us in one of the empty classrooms. When I finally explained to them that what was causing her headaches was "constipation," they were surprised. I never read again that she was having headaches, but I was disappointed because neither she nor her mother ever thanked me for helping. It makes you wonder if they appreciated this help.

You may contact Dr. Schulze's American Botanical Pharmacy by calling 1-800-HERB-DOC. He will be glad to send you a catalog as well as his news letter and also to fill your order. You may want to order Intestinal Formula # 1, Intestinal Formula # 2, Echinacea Plus, Cayenne Tincture, SuperFood, etc. As I have said before, I highly recommend his treatments as this may solve most of your health problems.

HOW YOU MAY STOP LOSING YOUR HAIR

Take the following daily:

1. SAW PALMETTO

2. PYGEUM

(Note: Men, 1 and 2, plus 30 mg of zinc each day may help your prostate. I know it works for me.)

3. L-CYSTEINE

4. VITAMIN B-6 (100 mg per day)

5. VITAMIN D (5000 i.u. per day- Note: I've read that zinc destroys some of your vitamin D. This is probably why you need 5000 i.u. per day.)

6. VITAMIN A (5,000 i.u.)

7. HORSETAIL

8. SILICA

Remember, nothing you take for your loss of hair will work in a hurry. Be patient.

Chapter Thirteen

Garlic and Other Cures

GARLIC MAY CURE YOUR CANCER

I just read a letter from an attorney in Houston, TX whose name is Smith and who cured his cancer. He ordered and read a booklet on garlic and states that he has long believed that garlic had many healing powers.

He decided to try a body cleansing program, which consisted of using three cloves of raw garlic each day. He claims he obtained remarkable results. Although he states that he has been a vegetarian for many years, he was surprised to find that in his stools there were worms- pin worms, round worms, and flat worms. He was shocked to find that everyone has long known that a great way to get rid of your worms is with garlic. He encountered only one real problem. After he had used the garlic for slightly over a week, his wife became extremely distressed because of the awesome smell that she wouldn't have anything to do with him.

My suggestion is if you decide to try this treatment, for you to use an empty cabin in the woods that belongs to some friends, or rent a hotel room and stay in it alone for about 10 days for your treatments.

Garlic may be one of the few ways to get rid of some forms of cancer, such as cancer of the brain. I know there is a lady in Europe who treats her cancer patients by using garlic. She requires everyone who comes into her sanitarium to eat garlic before entering, including herself. Apparently this low cost treatment is very effective.

We know that the ingredient in garlic which helps us so much is allicin. We can take the "social garlic" which is not supposed to give any odor until it is in our intestines, but it is not nearly as effective as the raw garlic. I have eaten the raw garlic and find it to be palatable. I would certainly recommend it for your cancer if you want an inexpensive, very effective, and very positive treatment which is extremely likely to cure your cancer.

The parasites can't stand the smell and will leave your body by the millions or even by the billions until you are virtually free of all parasites.

THE SALT TREATMENT MAY CURE YOUR CANCER

Once there was a man in Mexico whose wife was dying of cancer. He had spent lots of time investigating salt and salt-restricted diets of other cancer patients, and he spent much time reasoning with his wife. He had spent much time talking with many terminal cancer patients who were coming and going from the same hospital his wife had attended. THEY WERE ALL TOLD NOT TO USE ANY SALT! No reason was given and I certainly know of no valid reason for this. The husband reasoned that if all these people who are dying of cancer are restricted from salt, surely his own wife would die also, so why not try using salt to see if it will make a difference? His wife agreed to the experiment and ate three tablespoons of salt the first day, two the second day, and then gradually she took less and less as each day she began to revive and feel much better. FINALLY HER CANCER WAS GONE, AND SHE IS STILL LIVING! The salt the Mexican man gave his wife was rock salt, commonly known to us as ice cream salt. I bought some myself after reading this. Read on for more information on how to use salt for treating your cancer. (Note: Feed stores sell rock salt in 50 pound bags and you may also buy it from other places. If you want to order this without having to hunt for a store that sells it, I recommend buying it from N.A.T.R. of California, 2806 Broadway, Suite 2, Dept. 7, Eureka, CA 95501. 770-442-4716.)

A man named Forrest Smith wrote the following: "From this story I put up a little experiment where I demonstrated at a recent health lecture, I set up three glass quart fruit jars. I took three kinds of salt, regular salt from the grocery store, sea salt from the health food store, and rock salt. I filled the jars with filtered water and put one teaspoon full of each type of salt in each jar and stirred until dissolved. Two jars looked very cloudy while the rock salt water was as clear as could be. The reason is that the two salts sold for human consumption had aluminum tricilicate in them to prevent the salt from caking. At that demonstration I put about a half cup of rock salt in a little whizzer and in just four or five seconds whizzed it to salt shaker granules. By adding some rice or a few beans to the salt shaker the ground rock salt, which tends to cake, can be quickly broken up with a few shakes.

You can rest assured that from now on we only use rock salt in our home. It tastes better and we know we won't end up with aluminum shorting out our brains when we get older. That malady is going around you know. We take a few kelp tablets (from the health food store) to provide iodine in our diet because rock salt is not iodized.

I recently learned that a friend was at home and very ill with shingles, and not doing well at all. I telephoned him and sure enough he was not doing well at all. I ended up by telling him about my own experience years ago with stomach ulcers, and how I, because of the testimony of a friend, had decided to try this crazy salt water cleansing treatment that was supposed to help anybody with any type of trouble. (Note: The exception to this rule is people with salt-free diets, edema, or heart trouble.) A friend of mine and I stopped at a famous health spa to check it out. I was not about to drink hot salt water to cleanse my stomach and bowels because I regularly had three bowel movements each day, but this determined buddy of mine finally talked me into taking it.

At that time, with my stomach trouble, I was living on buttermilk, soft boiled eggs, jello, and milk toast. It made me sick if I ate vegetables or fruit, and with this bland diet, I often had to lie on my stomach to get relief. I really needed a stomach and bowel cleansing, but didn't know it. The owner of the health spa told me that after I cleansed with salt water, I could then (for breakfast) eat all the fruit I wanted and it wouldn't hurt me. I didn't believe him. He also said before I took the salt water treatment although, if I ate any beans, I would be sick in bed with a fever for a day or two, but after the salt water treatment, he indicated that I could eat beans and not get sick. I did not believe this either.

Since I had taken the salt water treatment, I decided to find out if this health spa owner was crazy or correct. I went through the cafeteria line and loaded my tray with fruit, and waited for the ill effects, but they never came. I still found this hard to believe.

On the way home, I bought several lovely peaches. At breakfast, my wife saw me eating a peach and she raised her voice in protest, knowing that I would be ill. I just smiled and kept on eating the peach. Finally, I broke down and told her about the salt water treatment and how I now could eat anything. When she cooked beans a little later on, I ate all I wanted and I've been eating them ever since.

When either of our children got a cold, I encouraged our child to take the salt water treatment. Their colds didn't amount to very much, and, when you get a cold, this is the body's effort to cleanse itself. When we cleanse with salt water, there is little need for the body to cleanse itself. So our colds don't last very long and normally won't happen if a person cleanses regularly with salt water.

We have also learned that if a person has diarrhea, if he cleanses with the salt water, the diarrhea stops. We have also learned that if a person has headaches, or bad breath, both will go away with the salt treatment.

It is a good idea to take the salt water treatment about twelve times per year. You won't need it so often in the summer as in the winter. If you have been exposed to a bad cold, flu, or pneumonia, you should take the cleansing the next day, or sooner. It is always best to prevent sickness than to treat if after the fact.

Most people suffer with constipation, although they don't realize it. A man went to his doctor because he was feeling bad. After the doctor checked him over, he was told that he was constipated. The man replied that this was not true as he had three bowel movements per day. The doctor replied, "All right, then you take these dozen grains of yellow popcorn and swallow them like pills with your dinner tonight. Then you watch your stools and call me when they have passed. The man called his doctor twelve days later to state that they had passed. We know that the residue of food we eat today should pass within 24 hours. When it doesn't, it tends to putrefy. Different diseases are able to develop and are permitted to take hold of us because of our dirty large intestine tracts. Getting rid of junk foods, cheap foods, rotting foods, etc is a real challenge to our digestive system. The best thing that anyone ever did for my health was to introduce me, to persuade me, to take the salt water cleansing.

Now I need to go back to my business friend with shingles. He had asked when and how he could take the treatment. He ended up taking it two days in a row BUT NEVER HAS A BOWEL MOVEMENT. While this is very unusual, it is nevertheless normal if your body needs salt. Normally the salt water flushed the bowels very well several times, but if the body is low on salt, or if a person is anemic, no bowel movement will occur until the treatment is taken for the third day.

However, the good news is that my business friend was very happy because he was coming back to life again. He is doing very well now-his body needed sodium chloride.

Recently, my wife has been complaining about phlem in her throat every morning which bothers her when she makes phone calls. This has been giving her trouble for months. I gave her a plastic cup with some rock salt in it and suggested that she dissolve a piece or two of it in her mouth. It stopped her trouble immediately. Why? I don't know, but maybe she needed some salt minerals.

HOW TO TAKE
THE SALT WATER TREATMENT

Before I tell you how to take the salt water treatments to cleanse the G.I. tracts (Gastrointestinal tracts), I need to tell you a story.

You may hear about the danger of a person getting too much salt. You may even read in a newspaper article about someone being saved from drowning in the ocean, who afterwards died because he drank too much salt water. There is both truth and error in such a report, in my opinion. Yes, he died, but it was not the salt water that killed him, BUT IT WAS HIS OWN ACCUMULATED POISON IN HIS G.I. TRACT that killed him. The salt water flushed it loose, but there was not enough water with it to flush it out. The average person's G.I. tract develops pockets which seldom, if ever, get emptied and as a result, poison is manufactured there. This is due to the following: improper diet, demineralized food, grease, sugar, junk food, lack of exercise, lack of high fiber food, lack of water, lack of minerals, eating between meals, eating too much protein, eating too late at night, not allowing a full five hours between meals, drinking liquid with the meal, and eating too much cooked food. The body then sheilds itself from these poisons and holds them there. If you were to go to a place in your city where they do colonic bowel irrigations, (there is normally one or more in each city) you will be able to see for yourself the stuff that is flushed from the bowels, and there will come out long strips of black, hard, rubber-like stuff that has the corrugated shape of your colon. Don't think you aren't affected, as nearly everyone is. But because there is a lot of water with the poison, it is flushed out and there is no harm. If you should become a terminal cancer patient and go south of the border for your health treatments, you would find that cleansing of the bowels is basic. Poison and filth in our colons are our number one health problem.

You are probably saying that heart trouble is our number one health problem. This is incorrect, because heart trouble is a last symptom. Poisons in our G.I. tracts is America's number one health problem, and nearly all diseases, including cancer, can be attributed to poison and filth in our colons. If you can show me a person who has for years kept a clean colon, he won't have cancer or heart trouble.

Once there was a lady who nearly died of candidiasis, a yeast infection, who had to get an education to save her own life. After that, she began helping others. She is a registered colonic specialist now. At her place of treatment, she always examines any bowel residue caught in the screen for each patient. The residue is thoroughly washed and disinfected before being brought to her for examination. Over the years, she has learned that flushing the bowels four days in a row is much more beneficial than three days. Because she always noticed a definite benefit for the fourth day, she always recommends a four day colonic program.

HOW TO USE
SALT WATER FOR CLEANSING

1. You should only take it on an empty stomach first thing in the morning. After the evening meal digests at night, the eleseekol valve in your colon opens and rests until any food or food drink, including tea or juice, is taken. As soon as anything besides plain water is taken, this valve closes. However, it does not close for salt water. (Note: Salt water, especially clean ocean water, can be used for blood transfusions. The analysis of sea water and blood is almost identical, so if any of my family ever needs a blood transfusion, I'll settle for clean sea water. A naval officer in World War II was about dead from loss of blood. They used four liters of sea water and he did very well.)

When sea water is taken first thing in the morning, it goes right on through to cleanse the bowels, and the results are not like taking a drug store laxative. Laxatives move the bowels, but do not carry away all the toxic material. Consequently, the body picks up new toxic poison and leaves a person feeling punk. With the salt water cleansing, there is enough water to flush it all out and it leaves one feeling like a million dollars. There have been a very few whose colons were so extended and full of unnecessary constipation that they never had a bowel movement and felt stuffy. In that case, they should get to the bottom of the problem with an enema, and start the works moving.

2. We take two quarts of the salt water for a treatment. A person's stomach will hold a quart. Always take two full quarts, and never stop with just one. In a quart of drinkably hot water, not too hot, add two teaspoons of salt. It's best to drink it quickly and get it over with, and this will give a better bowel action. About ten minutes after drinking the first quart, I mix the salt in the second quart and drink it one glass at a time within the next ten or fifteen minutes. If possible, both quarts should be taken within about 30 minutes. Then when Mother Nature says go, you don't ask "what did you say?," you obey. Most people find that a little mentholatum on the anus protects it from caustic toxins that the salt water will flush out.

3. The way to mix is to use two rolling teaspoons of salt to each quart of hot water. The way to keep from getting the water too hot is to test the water first, then add the salt and stir until dissolved. Drink the first quart right down, and, of course, USE ONLY ROCK SALT, no more aluminum.

4. We make it a habit of eating only some juicy fruit or melon or drinking juice for breakfast after the treatment, but that is not necessary. As much water or liquid as one can take that day is essential and here is why. When the poisons and bad accumulations in the colon are flushed away, the body then is generally relieved and there is now reason and room to let go of other toxins it has been covering and putting up with, and naturally it requires liquid to do that. So, be sure to take in plenty of liquids on that day.

HOW YOU MAY ADD YEARS TO YOUR LIFE

We don't have a family doctor now; we don't need one since we learned of the salt water treatment. Several friends and I talked a 64 year old man who was very ill and waiting to get well, so he could begin his three operations his doctor had lined up for him, into taking the salt water treatment. He took the treatment and, as a result, never had to have any of his three operations.

Babies who get pneumonia and about to die, have been brought right out of it by giving them a bottle of this salt water. People with migraine headaches have forgotten that they ever had a headache, and people with ulcers now eat anything. People with bad breath are now pleasant to talk to. People who didn't know what their trouble was, and neither did the doctors, now feel fine, and they know what to do if they start to feel bad again. Unless a person has edema, or heart trouble, or is restricted from salt, the salt water treatment is the first thing we think of. It isn't a cure at all, but it is basic, we believe.

The person who invented this salt water cleansing says that it will add 10-15 years to a person's life. This is easy to believe because he introduced it to many people who were in bad health and about ready to give up, who snapped out of it and lived many more years. He knows people who were on their last leg, and by keeping their colons clean, are still hanging in there. He has a picture of an 87 year old man with his 7 year old son, who takes a colon cleansing often. Does that tell you anything?

In our opinion, people in general would benefit greatly by taking at least 12 salt water cleansings a year. For something serious (like cancer), four mornings in a row followed each time by lots of juice.

This man John, whom we met that was not doing well and who was trying to get well so that he could start the first of three operations his doctor had lined up for him, decided to take the salt water treatment along with myself and several friends. There were several homes close together that summer day, and we all took the treatment that day together on the lawn under the shade of several lovely cedar trees. We all drank down our first quart, and in about five minutes we started drinking our second quart. NEVER STOP WITH ONE QUART as it takes two quarts to provide enough water to do the flushing properly. We all finished our second quart within about 25 minutes. My new sick friend John, suddenly excused himself and went aside and regurgitated the second quart he had just taken. I KNEW WHAT THE PROBLEM WAS. HIS STOMACH WAS SO LOADED WITH TOXIN, THAT HIS BODY KNEW THE CLOSEST AVENUE TO GET RID OF IT. When he settled down, I patted him on the back and said, "Well John, you lost a quart, but we'll give you another one to take its place." This probably surprised him, but he drank another quart and this time it stayed down. Two weeks later, we met John again and he was a different man, as he was not sick anymore. I asked him if he had taken the salt water treatment anymore, and he said that he had not. He further stated that he was not going to have any of those operations, and he is going to all of his friends in the Bay Area and wants to teach them how to get well and how to stay well. We have never seen John again, but I'm certain that his testimony and influence has probably helped many people who were suffering.

MIGRAINE HEADACHES

Susan was 34 years old and the perfect picture of health, but as I talked to a small group of people, she spoke up and said, "I'm in perfect health, but I have terrible migraine headaches every afternoon for about 5 hours. I've been to many doctors but none can help me." I replied that I believed that her headaches were coming from her body feeding on toxins (poisons) in her colon. She took the salt water treatment that next morning, and that afternoon she came to my house and reported that she had not had her daily headache. Two weeks later, she came to my home overjoyed that she had not had any more headaches. Just from that one treatment, I asked. She replied, "Yes, and I want to thank you from the bottom of my heart."

ONLY 30 DAYS TO LIVE

One of my very close friends, who used to work with me, phoned me from Washington State not long ago. His medical doctor there had informed him that he had cancer of the pancreas and had 30 days or less to live. He asked me what he could take, what I would suggest. I told him that if his doctor told him he had 30 days, or less, to live, he had only one shot at this cancer and better forget even the self-treatments that are known to be effective against cancer. If it's the wrong shot, you lose. He agreed and asked what I would do. I unhesitatingly suggested Hospital Santa Monica, across the border out of San Diego 619-428-8585 (1-800-767-8585 for out of California, toll free.) It's a nice new hospital, and when you get there, you know you are among friends who care.

We know when your pancreas goes, you go with it. He may have had only a few days to live and if I had suggested treatments I knew might heal him and still if he died because he didn't have enough time for the treatments to be effective, I would have felt that I failed him. The good news is he made it because he went to Mexico and received the best possible treatments.

The next question is WHY DID HE GET CANCER? My opinion is that he got cancer BECAUSE HE DID NOT KEEP HIS COLON CLEAN. The human body can take a lot of punishment, but when the G.I. tract is not bathed once in a while, disease may develop. This friend, by the way, was a strict vegetarian for over 30 years, was a hard worker, and was not overweight. The news of his bout with cancer shocked everyone. My opinion is that he, like the rest of us, needed to bathe the inside as well as the outside. Please think it over. We bathe the outside daily, so why not the inside once in a while?

MELANOMA

Another friend of mine phoned me several years ago and said that he had a big melanoma on his neck and he didn't want to let the doctors touch it, and asked me for a phone number where he could get some hope. I suggested Hospital Santa Monica, under the direction of Kurt Donsback. Why do you suppose I suggested Hospital Santa Monica? At Hospital Santa Monica there was a case history which took place only a few days before my wife and I went there on a tour. A lady who had arthritis so bad in her hands and wrists that they were swollen up like clubs, very painful and no one could touch them. She had to be waited on. Dr. Donsback invented an intravenous infusion of minerals, non-toxic chemicals, vitamins and food grade hydrogen peroxide. The treatment takes three hours. Dr. Donsback was giving this lady the treatment and 45 minutes into the treatment, she began to sob. Dr. Donsback was concerned because the normal response is that it makes people feel great. He began to quickly try to find out where she hurt. Finally, she was able to say, "Oh no, doctor, I don't hurt but look, I can move my fingers." The very next day, 24 hours later, she went around and shook hands with over a hundred people in that hospital.

Yes, she was cured of her arthritis, and so was Walter Grotz, the retired postmaster that now lectures all over the world and tells how he was cured of his terrible arthritis for less than $6.00. Walter Grotz, had listened to Reverend Richard Welhelm talk about the benefits of food grade hydrogen peroxide taken internally in a dilute solution. Walter Grotz thought that this lecture was "wacky" but he kept listening and finally decided that it wouldn't hurt him, so he bought a bottle and started taking it. He doesn't have arthritis any longer.

WHAT CAUSES ARTHRITIS?

Basically arthritis is caused by anaerobic bacteria (bacteria that cannot live in oxygen, and thus, seek to live in areas within the joints where there is no blood.) Hydrogen peroxide enters the lymph system tissue, kills the anaerobic bacteria, and then the body can eliminate the excreted calcium which the bacteria deposited.

THE WORLD'S GREATEST DOCTOR

BACK TO MY FRIEND WITH MELANOMA

He hopped a plane from Texas to San Diego. The hospital van picked him up and took him across the border into Mexico. Thirteen days later he phoned me from Hospital Santa Monica and said that he had only been on the treatment for 11 days and you could hardly see the melanoma (and it had been about the size of an egg.) He just wanted to thank me for that phone number where he did get hope- and complete healing with natural, harmless, non-toxic methods. That was over three years ago, and I recently talked with him by phone, and he is still well.

WHY DID HE GET CANCER?

Again, here is the case of a strict vegetarian, over 35 years of careful eating, who got cancer. Why? Well, to me, it's the same old story, he did not make it a habit to cleanse the colon. I'm telling you, in my opinion, most all diseases and sickness stem from contamination in the colon. TAKE A BATH INSIDE. If disease is "an effort of nature to correct conditions that have been caused by the wrong habits of living," and that's exactly what it is, THEN CLEAN OUT GRAND CENTRAL STATION WHERE DISEASE STARTS.

INDIUM- THE MISSING TRACE MINERAL

This trace mineral was first patented for nutritional use in 1980, and its many users report life changing benefits. Indium may be good for a large number of ailments, and among them are the following: headaches, eye pain, runny nose, mouth sores, mouth ulcers, nausea, intestinal and bowel problems, depression, dizziness, sneezing, sinus pressure, sore throat, urinary problems, menstrual problems, and many others, including numerous forms of cancer.

Indium is non-toxic when taken orally in amounts recommended. We know that it is a trace mineral since it appears in very small amounts in the earth's crust. Indium is inorganic and our bodies cannot handle inorganic minerals. They must be made into a water soluble sulfate form. Even though we are unable to receive indium from the soil, our bodies still need it. Although it is not required for life, it is required for our health.

A man had a tumor of the rectum and the doctor used indium octreotide very effectively. This resulted in a great decrease in the size of the tumor and all symptoms soon disappeared. It has been successfully used on pancreatic cancer (which is one of the most deadly cancers), carcinoid tumors, and lung cancer. It has been determined that indium seeks out and destroys tumor tissue.

Normally indium sulfate as well as indium octreotide is taken in liquid form. Indium sulfate is the stronger of the two, and one drop is equal to 10 milligrams and is usually taken on an empty stomach (normally about 8 hours from the last bite). You put the drop on top of your tongue before anything else is taken and wait at least 30 minutes before eating anything. You continue for a month taking only one drop each morning. Whether or not you increase this to two drops per day or decrease it to one drop every other day depends on how you feel. Check with the manufacturer's or supplier's recommendation for this. There are numerous benefits to be obtained from use of indium sulfate or indium octreotide. It has been reported to help Parkinson's sufferers to improve their walking and speech in as little as two weeks. It is known to improve prostate gland health, and to extend the lifetime of red blood cells. There are numerous other benefits to be obtained from this trace mineral and of course you will want to determine all of its possible benefits and also to know if it is safe. Yes, it is very safe, and it has been determined that it would have to be over 1,000 times stronger than it is to even make a mouse sick. Since most trace minerals are not safe like this, this is the exception. It has a clean, strong tart taste and you will be able to taste it even though you only put one drop on your tongue. Although it normally takes slightly over a week for people to notice benefits from this, it affects the glands of takers during the first day.

I ordered a 90 day supply of this for $89.00 plus $4.95 shipping fees by telephoning 1-888-374-2363 and ordering item IN-XL 90 Day Supply of Micro-Drop Indium XL in dropper vial from East Park Research, Inc., 2709 Horseshoe Dr., Dept. 7, Las Vegas, NV 89120. The price is now $39. For 1 bottle or $78 for 3.

CAYENNE MAY CURE YOU

Dr. John Christopher was a great herbalist until he died. He was one of the all-time great doctors and contributed some great ideas for healing. He may have been too great for his own good as his success rate for healing was extraordinary. His fellow naturopathic physicians warned him that he was curing too many diseases, and doing it too fast. When he failed to heed their warning, he was arrested and sent to jail as a felon. They actually put him out of business because he was too great. How's that for justice in this country?

Dr. Christopher says that when he was 35 years old, his doctors told him that he would never live to see 43. He had advanced hardening of the arteries, and suffered from crippling arthritis, stomach ulcers, and he had also been involved in a very bad auto accident in which he suffered serious injuries. He was unable to buy life insurance, even $1,000 of it, as he was such a bad risk. When he turned to cayenne pepper, he says it saved his life. He started taking cayenne pepper three times per day in hot water, and did this for 10 years. His blood pressure became normal, and all of his health problems vanished. When he reached 45, he applied for a $100,000 life insurance policy and bought it. Of course, he passed the physical with flying colors.

To the best of my recollection, he was injured in an accident at home and died from head injuries when he was age 82. He was truly one of the all time great doctors and left us much great information to use for healing ourselves. Some of it is to follow now.

CAYENNE IS GREAT FOR STOPPING BLEEDING

One day two young boys were playing cops and robbers with their father's guns and the guns were unfortunately loaded. One of the children shot the other in the abdomen and the bullet hit the spine and ricocheted and made a second wound leaving the body. One of Dr. Christopher's students lived in the neighborhood and heard the shot, and rushed over to investigate. He knew the parents were away, and that the kids should not be shooting guns. The ten year old child was gushing blood from both his sides, and the neighbor ran to his cabinet and mixed some cayenne in a glass of water. He then poured it down the boy's throat and called for an ambulance.

When the boy arrived at the hospital he was the center of attention, not because of his wounds, but because he was not bleeding. One thing Dr. Christopher says is that "by the time you count to ten, cayenne will stop the bleeding." The doctor told the boy's parents that he had seen numerous accident victims in his lifetime, but this was the first time he has opened up an abdomen to find no blood, except for a minute amount that was there before the bleeding was so quickly stopped.

Dr. Christopher often used cayenne tincture directly on open wounds to stop the bleeding. Although this may sting a little, it does stop the bleeding promptly.

CAYENNE MAY SAVE YOU IF YOU HAVE A HEART ATTACK

Dr. Christopher believed that cayenne was one of the very finest foods for the heart and stated that he had been called numerous times over the years for heart attack cases, and each time cayenne saved them. He even claimed that in 35 years of treating heart attack patients, he had never lost one when he used cayenne. He said that when he arrived, if they are still breathing, he would pour down their throat a cup of cayenne tea. Within minutes, they would normally be up and around. He said that most heart patients were suffering from malnutrition because of the processed foods we eat, and he found cayenne to be the fastest acting acids he could possibly give the heart patient. Cayenne feeds the heart immediately.

CAYENNE MAY GET RID OF YOUR HIGH BLOOD PRESSURE

Dr. Christopher met an athlete whose mother had died from high blood pressure. He also had high blood pressure and it was getting worse. He noticed that Dr. Christopher took cayenne tea each morning and decided to try it himself. Sure enough, soon his blood pressure returned to normal and has stayed that way ever since, and he also got rid of his hemorrhoids from taking cayenne.

CAYENNE MAY HEAL YOUR BRAIN CANCER ALSO

Although the patient had terminal brain cancer, he decided that he only wanted to take one thing for it, and this was cayenne. His brain tumor was malignant, and his diagnosis showed that it was rapidly advancing. The doctors had told him that with this tumor, even with surgery, that he would only have a 5% chance of survival, so this probably caused him to decide that he would use only cayenne. He was warned that if this was all he would do to get rid of his cancer, he would have to take large doses of cayenne. He agreed to this, and after 45 days of massive doses of cayenne, his tumor was totally dissolved.

L-ARGININE

This amino acid is a very important one for all of us. When we take L-arginine, it supplies nitrogen, which is used to create nitric oxide from oxygen and nitrogen. It will help us men to obtain penile erections. It lowers our blood pressure so this makes it great for treating our high blood pressure also. Because it lowers our blood pressure, it helps us to obtain good erections. It actually enhances dilation of our arteries.

Approximately 3 grams of L-arginine may restore sexual functions in over 40% of users, although some men may need larger doses. Eighty percent of our semen is composed of L-arginine, so this makes this doubly important to us. It is also known to improve growth hormone release, wound healing, immune system functions, and helps to increase the strength of the heart muscles. It is generally considered safe up to 6 grams per day. Although it is a food substance, if you have diabetes, herpes, or cancer, you may need to consult your doctor before taking it.

I like L-arginine powder, so I buy the NOW brand and put one half teaspoon of it in some water, stir it, and take on an empty stomach. Ladies may take it for high blood pressure and also to help their sexual function.

It may take several weeks for you to get the reaction you desire from this L-arginine, so be patient.

Chapter Fourteen

Non-Toxic Therapies and Diagnostic Tests Directory

The following information was furnished courtesy of Cancer Control Society and is furnished for informational purposes only.

LAETRILE THERAPY

(Also known as Vit. B-17 or Amygdalin)

Robert Rowen, M.D.
615 E. 82nd Ave. #300
Anchorage, AK 99518
917-344-7775

American Biologics Hosp. Mexico   (U.S. Contact)
Robert & Carole Bradford, Founders   1180 Walnut Ave.
Playa De Tijuana, Mexico   Chula Vista, CA 91911
                                         619-429-8200
                                         800-227-4458

Harold Manner Memorial Hospital   (U.S. Contact)
Julian Mejia, M.D.   P.O. Box PMB 63
Tijuana, Mexico   439056
011-52-66-804422   San Ysidro, CA 92143
                                         800-248-8431
                                         888-281-6663

International BioCare Hospital   (U.S. Contact)
Rodrigo Rodriguez, M.D.   111 Elm St. #209
Tijuana, Mexico   San Diego, CA 92101
                                         800-785-0490

Oasis Hospital   (U.S. Contact)
Ernesto Contreras, M.D.   P.O. Box 439045
Playas De Tijuana, Mexico   San Ysidro, CA 92143
011-52-66-316100   800-700-1850

Stella Maris Clinic   (U.S. Contact)
Gilberto Alvarez, M.D.   P.O. Box 435123
Tijuana, Mexico   San Ysidro, CA 92143
011-52-66-343444   800-662-1319
                                         800-973-7909

Ruth Manner Walter, Spokeswoman (NY) 516-798-2888

METABOLIC THERAPY

Jesse Stoff, M.D.   Robert Roundtree, M.D.
IntegraMed Clinics   4150 Darley Ave. #1
2507 N. First Ave.   Boulder, CO 80303
Tucson, AZ 85719   303-499-9224
520-740-1315

Warren Levin, M.D.
13 Powder Horn Hill
Wilton, CT 06897
203-598-7400

Jeffrey Kerner, D.O.
200 Bassett Ave.
New Castle, DE 19720
302-328-0669

William Richardson, M.D.
ATL Clinic of Preventative Med.
1718 Peachtree St. N.W., #360
Atlanta, GA 30309
404-607-0570

John Toth, M.D.
2115 W. 10th St.
Topeka, KS 66604
785-232-3330

Paul Beals, M.D.
9101 Cherry Lane, #205
Laurel, MD 20708
301-490-9911
202-332-0370 (Washington D.C.)

James Around-Thomas, M.D.
220 Collingwood St.
Ann Arbor, MI 48103
734-995-4999

Ronald Schmid, N.D.
56 Fair Haven Dr.
Middleburn, CT 06762

Stephen B. Edelson, M.D.
Center for Environmental
& Preventative Medicine
3833 Roswell Rd., #110
Atlanta, GA 30342
404-841-0088

Ross Hauser, M.D.
Caring Medical & Rehab
Serv
715 Lake St., #600
Oak Park, IL 60301
708-848-7789

Charles Mary, III
1201 S. Clearview Pkwy.,
#100
Jefferson, LA 70121
504-734-0730

A. Shamim, M.D.
200 Fort Meade Rd.
Laurel, MD 20707
301-776-3700

Stephen Margolis, M.D.
37300 Dequindre Rd.,
#201   Sterling Heights,
MI 48310
810-268-0228

William Fierce, N.D.
9623-D E Independence Blvd.
Mathews, NC 28105
704-849-8266

Douglas Brodie, M.D.
601 W. Moana Lane, #3
Reno, NV 89509
775-829-1009

Ken Bock, M.D.
Rhinebeck Health Center
108 Montgomery St.
Rhinebeck, NY 12572
914-876-7082
518-435-0082 (Albany, NY)

Jack Slingluff, D.O.
5850 Fulton Rd. N.W.
Canton, OH 44718
330-494-8641

Howard Posner, M.D.
111 Balla Ave.
Balla Cynwyd, PA 19004
610-667-2927

Bolles Clinic
Betty Go, M.D.
15611 Bel Red Rd.
Bellevue, WA 98008
425-881-2224

Brian Briggs, M.D.
718 Sixth St. S.W.
Minot, ND 58701
701-838-6011

Robert Barnes, D.O.
3489 E. Main Rd.
Fredonia, NY 14063
716-679-3510

Michael Schachter, M.D.
2 Executive Blvd., #202
Suffern, NY 10901
845-368-4700

Donald Mantell, M.D.
589 Ekastown Rd.
Sarver, PA 16055
724-353-1100

Norman Saliba, M.D.
1630 S. Church St., #203
Murfreesboro, TN 37137
615-848-0113

Seattle Cancer Treatment
& Wellness Center
Mark Gignac, N.D.
901 Boren Ave., #901
Seattle, WA 98104
206-292-2277

Jim Chan, N.D.
101-3380 Maquinna Dr.
Vancouver, B.C., Canada V5S 4C6

Holistic Herb Health
Center
Ken Graw, Herbalist
R.R. 1
Wembley, AB,
Canada T0H 3S0
780-766-2021

Providence Pacifica Hospital
Gary Tarasov, M.D.
Tijuana, Mexico

(U.S. Contact)
2220 Otay Lakes Rd.,
#502-244
Chula Vista, CA 91915
619-972-3831

21st Century Medicine
Jose Mota, M.D.
Ave. Del Pacifico, #2641
Costa De Oro
Playas De Tijuana, Mexico
011-52-66-308192

New Hope Clinic
Bio Resonance Therapy Center
Tijuana, Mexico

(U.S. Contact)
416 W. San Ysidro Blvd.,
#301
San Ysidro, CA 92113
888-532-0897

Hospital Santa Monica
Kurt Donsbach, Ph.D.
Rosarito Beach, Mexico
011-52-66-313333

(U.S. Contact)
1227 3rd Ave.
Chula Vista, CA 91911
619-427-3007
800-359-6547

Hospital Baja Nor
Carlos Alensandrini, M.D.
Tijuana, Mexico
011-52-66-823005

(U.S. Contact)
P.O. Box 430531
San Diego, CA 92143

Frank Morales, M.D.
Rio Valley Medical Center
Matamoras, Mexico
011-52-88-124842

(U.S. Contact)
1424 W. Price Rd., #450
Brownsville, TX 78520
956-778-3329

Ricardo James, M.D.
Good Samaritan Med. Center
Juarez, Mexico

(U.S. Contact)
PMB #460
6001 Gateway West F-14
El Paso, TX 79925
915-727-4429
877-319-6510

Francisco Soto, M.D.
Advanced Medical Group
Juarez, Mexico

(U.S. Contact)
5862 Cromo Dr., #147
El Paso, TX 79912
800-863-7686

FOR LAETRILE (B-17)

(DMSO, Hydrazine Sulfate, Enzymes and Other Supplements)

Bio Research Institute
4492 Camino De La Plaza, #TIJ 1063
San Diego, CA 92173
011-52-66-305865
800-291-1508

Kem, S.A. Laboratories
482 W. San Ysidro Blvd.
#207
San Ysidro, CA 92173
800-851-9470

Great Expectations
P.O. Box 6888
Los Osos, CA 93412

Holistic Alternatives
9181 Baker Rd.
St. Louisville, OH 43071
740-745-5741

World Without Cancer, Inc.
1111 Kane Concourse #303
Bay Harbor Island, FL 33154
305-861-0685
888-301-1336

SUPPLEMENTS

American Biologics
1180 Walnut Ave.
Chula Vista, CA 91911
619-429-8200
800-227-4473

EcoNugenics, Inc.
2208 Northpoint Pkwy.
Santa Rosa, CA 95407
707-521-3370

Life Support
(POLY-MVA)
P.O. Box 4651
Modesto, CA 95352
209-529-4697

C.P.W. Rahlstedt
P.O. Box 730527
D-22125 Hamburg, Germany
011-49-177-2441314

APRICOT KERNELS

Sun Organic Farm
P.O. Box 2429
Valley Center, CA 92082
888-269-9888

CANCER TESTS
(Immuno-Diagnostic Urine & Blood)

Oncolab-AMAS Test
Samuel Bogoch, M.D.
36 Fenway
Boston, MA 02215
617-536-0850
800-922-8378

American Metabolic
Testing Labs
Emile Schandle, Ph.D.
1818 Sheridan St. #102
Hollywood, FL 33020
954-929-4814
954-929-4895

Healthexcel
(Nutritional Evaluation)
277 W. Chewuch Rd.
Winthrop, WA 98862
509-996-2131

Hospital Ernesto Contreras
P.O. Box 439045
San Ysidro, CA 92143

Navarro Medical Clinic
3553 Sining, Morningside Terr.
Santa Mesa, Manila 2806
Philippines
011-632-714-7442

Dietmar Schildwaechter,
M.D.
Sovereign Consultants
Int'l
P.O. Box 16602
Dulles Int'l Airport
Washington D.C. 20041
703-430-7789

Scientific Regeneration
Inst.
Calle Ensenada #393
Tijuana, B.C., Mexico
011-52-66-849231

(U.S. Contact)
847-359-3634 (Evenings)

BREAST THERMOGRAPHY

William Cockburn, D.C.
11695 National Blvd.
Los Angeles, CA 90064
562-699-7921

ALTERNATIVE THERAPIES FOUNDATIONS

Robert Bradford Research Institute
1180 Walnut Ave.
Chula Vista, CA 91911
619-429-8200
800-277-4458

Linus Pauling Institute
Oregon State University
571 Weniger Hall
Corvallis, OR 97331
541-737-5075

Int'l Bio-Oxidative Medicine
Foundation
P.O. Box 891954
Oklahoma City, OK 73189
405-478-4266

HYPERTHERMIA

(Microwave Hyperthermia combined with Radiation)

Valley Cancer Institute
12099 W. Washington Blvd. #304
Los Angeles, CA 90066
310-398-0013

Advanced Center of Integrated
Medicine
Jeffrey Freeman, M.D.
Tijuana, Mexico
011-52-66-824902

(U.S. Contact)
P.O. Box 926
Bonita, CA 91908
619-472-1588

CELLULAR THERAPY

American Biologics Hosp. Mexico
(Tijuana, Mexico)
1180 Walnut Ave.
Chula Vista, CA 91911
619-429-8200
800-227-4458

Dr. Miller Medica
Milcell-Resomillan
Ballindamm 11
2000 Hamburg 1,
Germany
011-49-40-324041

NUTRITION PROGRAM

James Privitera, M.D.
105 N. Grandview Ave.
Covina, CA 91723
626-966-1618

Davis Lamson, N.D.
Jonathan Wright, M.D
515 W. Harrison St #200
Kent, WA 98032
253-854-4900

GERSON THERAPY

Gerson Institute-Oasis
Charlotte Gerson, Founder
P.O. Box 430
Bonita, CA 91908

Hospital Meridien
Luz Bravo, M.D.
Tijuana, Mexico

Gerson Therapy
Self-Help
Marilyn Barnes Bloom
59-A Massolo Dr.
Pleasant Hill, CA 94523
800-851-8473

(U.S. Contact)
P.O. Box 489
Bonita, CA 91908
619-425-4625
877-329-4460

HOXSEY THERAPY
(Herbal)

Bio-Medical Center
615 General Ferreira
(Colonial Juarez)
Tijuana, B.C. Mexico
011-52-66-849011
011-52-66-849132 Evening

(U.S. Contact)
P.O. Box 433654
San Ysidro, CA 92173

IMMUNOTHERAPY
(Vaccines & Nutrition)

Immune Institute
Darrell See, M.D.
18800 Deleware St. #900
Huntington Beach, CA 92648
714-842-1777

Naima Abdel-Ghany, M.D.
340 W. 23rd St. #K
Panama City, FL 32405
850-872-8122

Issels-Gerson Cancer Center
Dan Rogers, M.D. CHIPSA
Tijuana, Mexico

Immunology Researching Center
Lawrence Burton, Ph.D., Founder
Freeport Grand Bahamas Island

American Metabolic Institute
Geronimo Rubio, M.D.
Tijuana, Mexico

Livingston Fdt. Med.
Center
3232 Duke St.
San Diego, CA 92110
619-224-3515

Burzynski Research Inst.
(Antineoplaston Therapy)
12000 Richmond Ave.
#260
Houston, TX 77082
281-597-0111

(U.S. Contact)
P.O. Box 1850
Chula Vista, CA 91212
858-573-9720 toll free
858-573-9721 fax
877-424-4772

(U.S. Contact)
P.O. Box 22579
Ft. Lauderdale, FL 33335
242-352-7455

(U.S. Contact)
555 Saturn Blvd.,
Bldg. B
M/S 432
San Diego, CA 92154
619-267-1107
800-388-1083

Institute of Chronic Disease
Gustavo Andrade, M.D.
416 W. San Ysidro Blvd. #677
San Ysidro, CA 92073
619-975-0216 pager

PREVENTION

Cancer Prevention Coalition
Samuel Epstein, M.D. Chairman
University of Illinois
School of Public Health
2121 W. Taylor St.
Chicago, IL 60612
312-996-2297
312-996-1374 fax

MAGNETIC THERAPY

William Philpott, M.D.
Research Consultant
17171 SE 29th St.
Choctaw, OK 73020
405-390-3009

WHEAT GRASS THERAPY

The Optimum Health Institute
6970 Central Ave.
Lemon Grove, CA 91945
619-464-3346

Ann Wigmore Institute
P.O. Box 429
Rincon, PR 00677
809-868-6307

Hippocrates Health Inst.
1443 Palmdale Ct.
West Palm Beach, FL
33411
561-471-8876

INSURANCE COORDINATORS

Health Insurance Claims Billing, Inc.
3033 Chimney Rock Rd. #620
Houston, TX 77056
800-843-6737

TRAVEL

CCS Cancer Clinic Tours
& Travel Service
P.O. Box 4651
Modesto, CA 95352
209-529-4697

Aeromedevac Air Ambulance
4420 Rainer Ave. #202
San Diego, CA 92120
619-284-7910
800-462-0911

Private Cancer Clinic
Tours
P.O. Box 530218
San Diego, CA 92153
619-475-3834

LOCAL HOTELS
(Shuttle Service Included)

Americana Inn & Suites
815 W. San Ysidro Blvd.
San Ysidro, CA 92173
619-428-5521
800-553-3933

Int'l Motor Inn/RV Park
190 E. Calle Primera
San Ysidro, CA 92173
619-428-4486

Chapter Fifteen

Dr. Clark

One of my clients telephoned me and just before he hung up the phone, he asked if I had read Dr. Clark's book. I asked him what the title of the book is and he said, "The Cure For All Diseases." He told me it was just absolutely great and that I should buy a copy.

Several more of my clients said the same thing, and I started wondering if this was really the great book my clients claimed. I finally decided to give in and buy a copy. The list price is $21.95, but to my surprise, three different vendors informed me that their price was $29.95. I was surprised inasmuch as I usually can buy at the list price or at a discount. Since I really wanted a copy, I finally broke down and paid them the inflated price.

Dr. Clark tells you how to make your own zapper, but I opted to buy one. She indicates that you put a nine-volt battery in the mechanism and turn it on. There are two copper polarity poles attached to two wires coming from inside the zapper, so you take a paper towel, tear it into two equal pieces, and wet both. After you squeeze out the excess water, you wrap one piece around each of these two copper polarity poles and turn on the zapper. It doesn't shock you, but it still has enough shock and voltage to kill the parasites by the millions. It won't kill the parasites in your heart, liver, kidneys, and other organs, but it will kill a gargantuan amount of these viruses and bacteria during the seven minutes you keep it turned on. So you turn it off for twenty to thirty minutes and then you use it twice more for seven minutes, with a twenty to thirty minute break each time, and you're through for the day. You have killed millions of parasites, and now don't have nearly so many left as you started out with.

"Why do you take these breaks?" you may ask. Parasites have parasites within them just as we do, so when you kill parasites, you don't kill those inside the parasites until they come out. They won't come out to be killed as long as you have the eliminator turned on, but will come out within a reasonable time after you turn it off.

I've been using my zapper for over three and a half years and have not had so much as a cold, or the flu. It surely is nice not to have to miss work because of a cold, flu or some other illness. In addition, by using the parasite eliminator, we aren't likely to contract pneumonia, or some other disease. One lady indicated that she was dying of lupus, and after she used her zapper for awhile, she returned to her doctor who did some tests on her. He was shocked at what he saw. He came out telling her that he was puzzled at the results of her tests because HER WHITE BLOOD CELLS HAD INCREASED IN NUMBER, whereas normally they decrease when you have lupus. He said that he had never seen this before. When she returned a month later, he told her that the results of the latest tests he had just done on her indicated that her white blood cells were normal and so was everything else. He could find no sign of the lupus. Hallelujah! She was well thanks to the zapper. In her book "The Cure For Advanced Cancers," Dr. Clark starts as follows: "If you have advanced cancer, you have no time to lose. You must accomplish three things with great haste to recover:

- stop the malignancy
- shrink the tumors
- remove the toxicity in your vital organs that leads to mortality.

If you have been given less than six months to live, go directly to the 21 Day Cancer Curing Program on page 179 of Dr. Clark's book. As soon as you are making progress, you can come back and read the explanations in the other chapters.

Also, read the case histories; see how hopeless the situation was and how simple it is to stop the cancer, shrink the tumor, and feel safe from ever having cancer again."

Dr. Clark indicated that one lady had a colonoscopy which seemed to indicate she was free of colon cancer, but when she had a test on the synchrometer a few days later, it indicated she had cancer. Dr. Clark then checked to see which part of her body had the cancer and to the patient's surprise, it was in her colon. When she went back to the people who did her colonoscopy, they found that they had made a horrible mistake because she did have cancer in her colon.

Hulda Regehr Clark, Ph. D., N.D., has written four books that I know of. In addition to "The Cure For All Diseases," she has written the following books: "The Cure For All Cancers," "The Cure For Advanced Cancers," and "The Cure For HIV and AIDS." In "The Cure For Advanced Cancers," she starts with the following: she has a 21-day cancer curing program set up for you to follow. It isn't easy to do but it is certainly not impossible. She follows this with information telling you how to read your blood test results, and how to improve on them in each area where you are too high or low. She tells you to keep on using your zapper each day to keep the cancer from spreading.

When I started reading the book, I got excited about it too. It indicated that all diseases are caused by just two things: parasites and pollution. Dr. Clark also indicated that you may kill parasites in your body by buying a zapper, which is a parasite eliminator.

All of her books listed above are excellent and I heartily recommend them. She has put a lot of work into these projects and is a very smart lady. You will definitely benefit if you use the zapper to help keep you well. You may read her book and make your own zapper. I know someone who has done this and he finds it to be very acceptable and helpful.

Chapter Sixteen

Vitamin Q

In most instances, this will probably be called CoQ10. I have no idea why this is called CoQ10 instead of Vitamin Q. This is a vitamin that is ubiquitous, which means it is found in every one of your cells. It is also called "ubiquinone." It is one of the greatest discoveries in nutrition of all time and unfortunately it has been sitting around undiscovered by almost everyone, including medical doctors.

Surprisingly enough, this vitamin has been around for over 35 years, yet almost no one knows anything about it. That's the way it is with vitamins because the doctors are slow to accept them and since they can't be patented, the drug companies and others will not spend any money to promote them. Remember, it took the doctors 200 years to accept vitamin C and to realize it is a great vitamin and could save your life. The reports about its treatment of cancer and heart problems are truly outstanding as you will see.

CANCER TREATMENTS

In all cancers with an adverse prognosis, the amount of CoQ10 levels are always low. You can actually determine if you will survive breast cancer, and probably other cancers, by determining the CoQ10 levels in your cells. The higher the CoQ10 level, the greater the chances of your winning the battle with cancer. If you get your CoQ10 levels in your cells up to a high level, you will increase your chances of licking cancer in any part of your body. If you want an ideal cancer treatment agent, you want one that will work along with the body and not against it. You want to strengthen your immune system, not destroy it. If you take chemotherapy or radiation, eventually you will destroy your immune system. Then you will be defenseless or almost defenseless if any disease comes along.

ONLY 25% OF CANCER VICTIMS DIE OF CANCER

In Dr. Hulda Clark's book "The Cure For All Cancers," she indicates that 25% of the cancer victims will die from the cancer, and 50% will die from heart problems or strokes.

CoQ10 is a great immune stimulator and also stimulates your blood system. Since it may take two or three months for your body to heal itself, you need to start taking this vitamin immediately. One good thing about taking this is there is no misery connected with taking it, and you will learn the meaning of real misery if you end up taking chemotherapy.

GETTING CoQ10

Since our bodies cannot manufacture this vitamin, we must buy it, although our bodies can make it if we take three other vitamins. If you will take Vitamin B3 (niacin), folic acid (also a B Vitamin), and pyridoxide (B6), your body will then be able to make CoQ10. You also need a combination of other vitamins, minerals, enzymes, amino acids, and cell salts to give your body what it needs. You should be able to find an excellent multivitamin tablet to take each day to give you most of what you need. One report says that the best form of CoQ10 to buy is manufactured by Vitaline and comes in a wafer form. I had to make a few phone calls before I was able to buy this. I had to call New York to get a large enough company that handled it, but at least I did succeed. According to this report, this form is best as it is one of the few that has been used in most of the past and present research throughout the world. The reason is that this CoQ10 has greater absorption over most other manufacturer's products. As you will see, there is another form of this vitamin which may be even better than the Vitaline.

TREATMENT RESULTS

Since I've got your attention, now it is the time to talk about results that we know about with this great vitamin. Dr. Karl Folkers, of the University of Texas gave the results of treatments of six cancer patients. Apparently some survived for five years and some survived fifteen years without any trace of cancer, and in five cases, the regression was total, and in the other case, there was regression of metastases in the liver, and the great thing about this form of treatment is there were never any side effects. (Note: Normally, a regression of metastases of cancer in the liver is fatal, but in this case, the cancer in the liver disappeared, and the patient recovered, thanks to Vitamin Q.)

The following are not testimonials but statements from doctors around the country in hospitals where a number of cancer patients were treated with Vitamin Q.

1. A 50 year old female with breast cancer had her right breast removed surgically to get rid of the cancer. A year later, the cancer was back. (Note by author: Actually I contend that all the doctor did was to remove a symptom, and not the cancer.) Since surgery was now impossible as her breast had already been removed, she was given x-ray treatments (sounds like radiation). A few months later, her doctor discovered that she had fluid in her right lung which also contained breast tumor cells. This meant she was without any hope for recovery. Then the doctor decided to try CoQ10, and started her on 90 milligrams per day, which was later changed to 390 mg per day. Six months later, her chest x-ray was normal and she had no sign of cancer. Three years later, she was still free of any symptoms of cancer.

2. A 40 year old female lost both breasts due to cancer and then took 10 treatments of three cancer drugs. An examination of her liver revealed metastases of her liver, which meant she was terminal. She was then given 390 mg of Vitamin Q per day and 12 months later, her metastases had disappeared, and she was in excellent health, with no cancer.

3. A 72 year old female developed cancer in her left breast and fortunately it had not spread. A lumpectomy was performed on her, but a microscopic examination showed that the cancer tissue had been cut through, causing the doctor to believe he had spread the cancer. A mastectomy was then performed. This patient had learned about CoQ10 and started taking it several months earlier at the rate of 100 mg per day. A full year later, her dosage was increased to 400 mg per day, and three years later she was still in good health, with no cancer.

With this, we would all wonder why aren't all cancer patients taking vitamin Q? It may take the doctors many years to accept this for treating cancer, and remember, it can't be patented, so it won't be advertised much, if any. The world will be slow to learn about it.

Although all of these cases were about breast cancer patients, this vitamin should work in all types of cancer. If you get every cell in your body at the optimum point with vitamin Q, it should strengthen your immune system enough so it can start destroying the cancer. If you can go for 5 years with no sign of cancer, I can't absolutely say that you are cured, but 10 years with no cancer, I would say you are free of cancer. One of the great side effects of loading your cells with vitamin Q so that your blood level of vitamin Q is close to three mcgs per cc of blood, is it will make you much healthier and may help you to fight not only cancer but all other diseases and health problems which may attack you. You will see how true this is a little later. Although this book is primarily about cancer, I see no reason why I shouldn't throw in other health areas which I know about that may be of interest to my readers.

After I learned about CoQ10, I started taking it and then I learned about the fact I should be taking the Vitaline, so I changed to this. I then started taking 320 mg per day plus consuming B3, folic acid, and B6 each day. I like 500 mg of B3, 800mcg of folic acid, and 500 mg of B6 per day, so this supplements the 320 mg per day I am purchasing and taking. (WARNING: If you take vitamin B3 (niacin), you may suffer a niacin flush. The first time my wife took vitamin B3, she called me from her school and told me she thought she was having a heart attack. After she told me about it, I told her she was having a niacin flush. If you want to avoid this niacin flush, take niacinamide instead.) I expect I was actually taking well over 400 mg per day, but don't actually know the exact amount. I predict that when doctors learn about this and start really prescribing it for patients, they may go as high as 600 mg per day for a seriously ill cancer patient, who may not have long to live. At least this may give the patient a chance to get well.

ANOTHER GOOD VITAMIN Q TO TAKE

The New England Heart and Longevity Clinic has been conducting some experiments and discovered a form of vitamin Q that has been scientifically proven to flood your body with up to 3 times more CoQ10 than typical tablets or capsules. They learned that CoQ10 gel, also called Q gel, was 3 times better than most of the other products. They claim that most formulations of CoQ10 are practically worthless. The reason is that some of their patients, who were taking 200 to 400 mg of CoQ10 daily, continued to have low levels of CoQ10 in their blood. They learned that the way most of their patients were taking CoQ10 was ineffective because this vitamin was passing right through their bodies unabsorbed. Under these circumstances, they might as well be throwing their pills down the toilet, because that is where much of the vitamin Q ends up. What we all need is the most absorbable form of vitamin Q.

ANOTHER VERY ABSORBABLE FORM

After they learned in 1997 that vitamin Q gel is up to three times more absorbable than typical CoQ10 tablets or wafers, this was proven by four separate lab tests, and their patients confirmed this because they started feeling so much better after they started taking the gel. Now, they have even improved on this. They learned that this vitamin works better if you take the Q-Gel TOGETHER with a nutrient called L-Carnitine.

WHAT IS L-CARNITINE?

L-Carnitine is a protein-like substance made in your liver and kidneys. (It's also an amino acid.) It works hand in hand with CoQ10 to provide your cells with maximum energy. Unfortunately, your supply of L-Carnitine declines as you age. I take 500 mg of L-Carnitine per day.

WHAT DOES L-CARNITINE DO THAT IS SO IMPORTANT?

L-Carnitine acts as a delivery system that brings needed nutrients to your body's cells. If these nutrients never make it to your cells, you have an energy shortage. Your heart has little "power plants" called mitochondria. The mitochondria are where your body turns food into energy.

On average, your heart cells contain 5,000 mitochondria, compared to only 200 mitochondria in each regular cell. This should give you an idea how much energy your heart needs.

There are different fuels your mitochondria uses to create energy. One fuel is CoQ10. This vitamin is the spark that helps increase your energy. Of all the organs in your body, your heart is the most responsive to CoQ10. That's because 10 times more CoQ10 is naturally found in your heart than anywhere else in your body.

Unfortunately, your body's CoQ10 production slows down as you age, and by the time you reach 40, you have 40% less vitamin Q than you had when you were 20. When you hit age 70, you will have 60% less, so this is why everyone over the age 40 needs to take CoQ10, and one of the best ways to take it is in the form of vitamin Q-Gel.

IS THERE ANOTHER FUEL THAT YOUR HEART NEEDS?

Yes. Your heart needs and loves essential fatty acids. In fact, essential fatty acids are responsible for 60-70% of your heart's energy. So, this is where L-Carnitine comes into play. It actually transports those fatty acids, the fuel, to your mitochondria, so without it your heart doesn't get the fatty acids it needs.

As we grow older, our liver and kidneys produce less L-Carnitine, so it becomes necessary to take it in supplemental form. This is why I recommend that you take L-Carnitine as well as CoQ10. If you take CoQ10 alone, you will miss out on lots of the benefits.

WHAT ARE THE BENEFITS BY TAKING THEM TOGETHER?

You will have a stronger heart, with healthy pumping action. I'm talking about healthy blood pressure, healthy cholesterol, and healthy triglyceride levels, as well as a metabolism that burns fat faster. I'm also talking about increased energy, and better well-being. This will help to keep your cells young and healthy, and may slow the aging process.

Patients who have taken both of these can't believe how much more energy they have and how much better they feel. They are then able to do things most of us take for granted, such as climbing a flight of stairs without being winded.

One patient named Joan had very little energy. Taking 180 mg of vitamin Q-Gel didn't seem to be helping her. She always felt very weak. Then the discovery of L-Carnitine came out and she started taking that also in the amount of 1000 mg per day. Her energy levels shot through the roof soon after that. I would also recommend that you take 100 mcg of vitamin B-12 each day also, besides the 800 mcg of folic acid, 500 mg of niacinamide (or B3), and 500 mg of pyridoxine (B-6). I also take 800 i.u. of vitamin E to help neutralize free radicals. It will be interesting to learn how much more it helps people with heart problems, Alzheimer's, Parkinson's disease and other diseases when the L-Carnitine and other substances recommended in this paragraph are added to the treatments.

WARNING:
BEWARE OF MIG BLASTS

Who is the MIG and why should they try to discredit the use of vitamins? The MIG is the medical-industrial governmental complex. There is no money in vitamins for the MIG, so they may do everything in their power to discredit the vitamin therapy. They hope they can steer you away from vitamins so that instead of taking vitamins, you will take drugs. We know that for any substance to be a drug, it must have one or more side effects. Quite often they have numerous side effects. I have seen some with as many as 23 side effects, and I have also seen them with a side effect such as THIS DRUG MAY KILL YOU! Would you want to take such a drug? Should your doctor make sure you know the risk when he prescribes a drug? I think he should, but they don't as they are not required to. Imagine if several of the drugs which were prescribed for you by your doctor were drugs which may kill you. I know of one patient who took 4 drugs in one day which could kill him, and he died that same day after taking them. If your doctor doesn't know all of the side effects, wouldn't you be afraid to take any drug? The only way to know if he knows the side effects is to ask him what they are. You can easily buy a book listing all of the side effects of drugs.

OTHER DISEASES

We know that eventually some of our doctors will get around to testing CoQ10 on numerous other diseases and we will learn the results. Since the CoQ10 used in testing has an enhanced absorption rate over other types of vitamin Q manufactured by others, it is able to cross the blood brain barrier. The blood brain barrier is difficult to get a nutrient to cross, so this would seem to give us a reason to hope it will be very effective in treating Alzheimer's disease as well as Parkinson's disease. There are undoubtedly numerous other diseases of the brain it may help.

HEART DISEASE

Surprisingly, CoQ10 is great for treatment of diseases of the heart. Heart failure is a great killer of the elderly, and it is increasing at an alarming rate. The baby boomers are getting to be elderly and will be joining in this undesirable increase in deaths due to heart problems. Here is a statement from one of the experts on vitamins: "Supplemental CoQ10 alters the natural history of cardiovascular illnesses and has the potential for prevention of cardiovascular disease...."

One of the first doctors to start treating patients with vitamin Q was Dr. Yuichi Yamamura in 1987 in Japan, which was 30 years after vitamin Q was discovered. His results were impressive but not enough to electrify the medical world, but at least it was a start.

Within our cells are little bodies called mitochondria, and they are the energy centers of our lives. CoQ10 is the fuel that runs our mitochondria engines. Without it, our atomic reactors cease to function. Our most important antioxidant would be lost, so we do need it.

Our hearts have one of the highest concentrations of vitamin Q of any part of our bodies. This should tell us of our needs for having lots of vitamin Q in our bodies. If you actually do have a high amount of CoQ10 in your heart, you can rest assured that you will probably live a long life into your 90s or 100s without a heart attack, or serious rhythmic abnormalities. Vitamin Q is probably the most important nutrient that you can take to have a healthy heart.

In a study on heart failures, in Japan, a large group of people with heart failures received treatments with CoQ10 and all of them improved, with over half showing no symptoms after only 4 weeks of treatments. We don't know what happened after this, nor do we know how much CoQ10 was given to them. In another study, 100 mg per day (this is a very small dose) caused a great increase in the survival rate of the heart patients. Normally, the survival rate would be less than ¼, but with only this small dose, after over 2 years, the survival rate was over 60%, even though these patients were seriously ill.

In cases where conventional treatments have failed, if the doctor will start giving the patients vitamin Q, great results often occur. In one case where the doctor had prescribed the standard treatment of water pills and digitalis, and when he realized it wasn't working, he gave all his heart patients CoQ10 in the amount of 100 mg per day. Over two thirds of the patients showed dramatic improvement objectively and subjectively after only 30 days. Surprisingly enough, this dose was totally inadequate from what we all know now. He should have given them 320 mg per day and probably all of them would have recovered.

In this experiment, they decided to try a new idea. They withdrew the vitamin Q from the patients who were doing so well and the patients went back to showing the same symptoms they originally had. Some had an increase in the heart rate, feeling lousy, liver congestion, shortness of breath, and swelling of the ankles. Then, they renewed the CoQ10 and their diets and these symptoms disappeared.

The problem with the treatments we know of so far is that it was too little and possibly too late. What would the results be if someone started taking 400 mg of vitamin Q at the start of the treatments? In still another test on well over 1,000 people, they only used 100 mg of CoQ10 for only 3 months, but still the results were great. Nearly 80%

of the patients showed great improvement in removing the symptoms and problems which were causing them to seek medical help.

IDEAS YOU MAY USE

You can contact a laboratory which makes blood tests and get them to test you for the amount of CoQ10 in your cells. If your level is low or if you have a heart problem, you may want to discuss this with your doctor and you might want to take 400 mg or even 600 mg of vitamin Q for a while and then have your blood checked again. When you reach a high level, you would then probably want to reduce the amount taken each day to 100 mg since you don't need large amounts. Hopefully, you will have good news for anyone who wants to know the results of the test you did. If you would like, please let me know about the results and what happened. I should like to hear from you. Write to me c/o the publisher of this book, and I will receive your letter.

CoQ10 now comes in a liquid form, which you administer by putting the drops under your tongue and keep it there for about twenty to thirty seconds and then swallow. The liquid form of this should also be very effective and give you quite a good dose of CoQ10. I know I tried it and liked it. It does not have a bad taste and is somewhat neutral as far as taste is concerned. You can find this in your local health food store.

LIVER KAMPO

If we look at longevity statistics, we know that Japanese people live longer than we Americans do. On average, Japanese women live five years longer than American women, and Japanese men live four years longer than American men. When we check to determine what caused this, we learned that an herbal medicine called Kampo has been around since 1866 and is regularly prescribed by doctors and is taught in half of the medical schools in Japan. They claim that Kampo may be used in treatments for upset stomachs, colds, treating liver disease, overcoming the effects of menopause, and it also INHIBITS THE GROWTH OF CANCERS.

It contains at least seven active ingredients, such as follows:

1. Pinellia tuber (increases interferon activity)

2. Scutellaria root (relaxes blood vessels, scavenges free radicals, reduces blood pressure, and EXHIBITS ANTITUMOR ACTIVITY)

3. Ginseng (INHIBITS CANCER CELL GROWTH BY SUPPRESSING THEIR DNS, and increases natural immune factors)

4. Jujube (an anti-asthmatic and INCREASES NATURAL KILLER CELL ACTIVITY)

5. Bupleurum root (reduces Parkinson's tremor, REDUCES ADHESION OF TUMOR CELLS AND ACTIVATES NATURAL DEFENSES AGAINST TUMOR CELLS)

6. Ginger (STOPS THE SPREAD OF CANCER CELLS)

7. Licorice (reduces Parkinson's tremor, is chemopreventive, protects your gastric system, and has antiviral activity)

Liver Kampo affects your complete body and it may be dangerous for you to take it if you are prone to develop colds often, flu or pneumonia. It is also dangerous to take it if you are taking tolbutamide, a drug for diabetes. If you take any type of diabetes medication, it may be dangerous to take Kampo because of the licorice therein. In any event, the sellers recommend you contact your doctor before taking Kampo if you have any health problems.

Even if you never buy Kampo, you may still use the above information to your advantage. You may start taking ginseng and ginger to kill cancer cells. If you wish to order Liver Kampo, you may do so by contacting Ben Salem Naturals, 371 Dartmouth Center, Dept 7, Bensalem, PA 19020, or telephone 215-638-0627. The cost is $22.91 per bottle plus shipping and handling for 180 tablets.

Chapter Seventeen

Spectro-Chrome

Dinshah P. Ghadiali lived in Bombay, India until he moved to America. While he lived in India, he was aware of the theory of chromopathy since he had studied the following books: "The Principles of Light and Color (1878)" by Edwin D. Babbitt, as well as "Blue & Red Lights" aka "Light & It's Rays as Medicine (1877)" by Dr. Seth Pancoast.

In the year 1897, he learned that a niece of one of his Theosophical Society friends was sent home by her doctor to die from a disease known as mucous colitis. He believed that her only hope for recovery lay in an unorthodox healing method, so he convinced her to try Dr. Edwin D. Babbitt's idea. He used the light from a kerosene lantern, with an indigo-colored glass bottle, which was used as a filter, and the light from this was shone on her. He took a milk bottle of the same color filled with milk and allowed the sunlight to shine on it for a while. She ultimately drank the milk to get the same benefits as when the light was used to cast the rays through the indigo bottle onto her body. She had an urgent need to evacuate and about one hundred times per day, she tried to do so. After just one day of treatments, she only had to make ten efforts to evacuate, and the treatments were so successful that she was able to get out of bed after only three days. This was the beginning of SPECTRO-CHROME, although it took him twenty-three years to give it this name.

In 1905, he was stricken with tuberculosis and only given six months to live by his medical consultant. He was advised to eat some meat, get plenty of rest and drink some wine for strength. He developed a number of treatments for tuberculosis, and probably healed himself because he had to do this to live. However, he refused to eat meat, or to drink wine, and actually got very little rest, and he still got well.

He left India in 1908 and in 1911 came to the U.S. with his wife and two children. In 1907, he became a citizen of the U.S. In 1920, he delivered his first lecture on Spectro-Chrome Therapy with 27 people present. He eventually taught at least 100 classes on this type of treatment. He even wrote books on Spectro-Chrome and in 1931 was charged with grand larceny- a complainant claimed he was defrauded by him because the plaintiff claimed that Spectro-Chrome could not have any effect on diseases. Dinshah proved that it did using a number of lay and medical practitioners to testify for him. (See the testimony of Dr. Kate Baldwin which follows.)

In 1924, he acquired 23 acres of property in Malaga, NJ, which then became the headquarters of the Spectro-Chrome Institute. In 1933, he wrote the Spectro-Chrome Metry Encyclopedia which is an authoritative treatise on color therapy. In 1941, he dissolved the Spectro-Chrome Institute and chartered the "Dinshah Spectro Chrome Institute" which is a non-profit corporation.

He had a number of setbacks in which he lost lawsuits and even had a six-week trial involving the FDA in which he was fined $20,000. All Spectro-Chrome books were ordered to be destroyed, although he was allowed to keep one copy and ordered to dissolve the Dinshah Spectro Chrome Institute and given 5 years probation. In 1953, he completed his probation and organized "The Visable Spectrum Institute," another non-profit corporation. The FDA obtained a permanent injunction against his new organization, which prevented shipment across state lines of color projectors and books pertaining to them. The injunction still stands today.

"Let There Be Light" is a wonderful book. I took 2 of the treatments listed in the book for my bleeding hemorrhoids and have had no further trouble with them. I have read numerous testimonials of people who claim to have received a cure for one or more diseases. As you can see from Dr. Kate Baldwin's testimony, many people claim to be cured using this type of treatment. Note: Dr Baldwin was the senior surgeon of the Women's Hospital of Philadelphia when she testified.

In May of 1930, Dinshah was arrested and jailed in Buffalo, NY and charged with "feloniously stealing $175 from Housman Hughes by falsely representing and PRETENDING THAT A CERTAIN INSTRUMENT AND MACHINE (Spectro-Chrome) would cure any and all human disease and ailments" etc. Now comes some of the trial testimony which includes a great deal of information about Spectro-Chrome.

THE TRIAL OF
MR. DINSHAH P. GHADIALI

The second witness was called by the Defendant and her name is Dr. Kate W. Baldwin. Her testimony follows:

DINSHAH- Where do you live?

BALDWIN- Philadelphia, Pennsylvania.

DINSHAH- Madam, what year did you graduate in Philadelphia, Pennsylvania?

BALDWIN- Medical College?

DINSHAH- In what year?

BALDWIN- 1890.

DINSHAH- You have been 40 years as an active physician?

BALDWIN- Yes sir.

DINSHAH- And your special line is surgery?

BALDWIN- Well, I am rated by the American College of Surgeons as a surgeon, as a Fellow by the American Academy of Ophthalmology and Oto-Laryngology; I have never confined myself, however, exactly to surgery.

JUSTICE- Forty-one years of general medical practice, is that right?

BALDWIN- Yes and surgery.

DINSHAH- You were the senior surgeon of the Women's Hospital of Philadelphia?

BALDWIN- Yes sir.

DINSHAH- How many years did you remain in charge of the surgical ward of the Women's Hospital of Philadelphia?

BALDWIN- I was the senior surgeon for 23 years. I had a clinic for almost the whole- for over 30 years, almost from the time I graduated, I was in clinical work.

DINSHAH- During the time that you were in charge of the surgical work, you performed numerous operations in surgery- major surgery?

BALDWIN- Pretty nearly everything from the crown of the head, to the soles of the feet.

DINSHAH- You are also a Fellow of the American Medical Association?

BALDWIN- Yes, sir.

DINSHAH- And a Life Member of the Maryland Academy of Sciences?

BALDWIN- Yes, sir.

DINSHAH- What other medical and scientific qualifications have you, madam?

BALDWIN- I don't know just what you mean.

DINSHAH- What other affiliations in medicine and surgery have you?

BALDWIN- Well, I belong to the County and State Medical Societies of Pennsylvania; I am also registered in Pennsylvania, New York and Rhode Island, to practice medicine and surgery. I had my intern's service at the Polytechnic Hospital, which is a good post graduate hospital. I also had clinical work in Boston, in the city hospital there and I belong to the American Academy of Ophthalmology and Oto-Laryngology. I was the first woman to be admitted to that organization. I am a member of the American College of Surgeons and of the American Medical Association, and various smaller societies, which perhaps you do not need to mention.

DINSHAH- Thank you. Now in your surgical work, in the Women's Hospital of Philadelphia- do I understand that the Woman's Hospital of Philadelphia is the oldest in the country?

BALDWIN- It is the oldest, women's hospital.

DINSHAH- It is the oldest, women's hospital. What year was it established?

BALDWIN- I cannot tell you.

DINSHAH- 1850?

BALDWIN- About that time.

DINSHAH- And you were in charge of the surgical work of that hospital for 23 years?

BALDWIN- Of the general surgery.

DINSHAH- Of the general surgery?

BALDWIN- Of the general surgical work; that did not include the gynecological surgery as far as the-

DINSHAH- General major surgery, really?

BALDWIN- General major surgery.

DINSHAH- Madam, how did you happen to meet me, the defendant at the bar?

BALDWIN- Some acquaintances of mine I met one evening and they said, "Doctor Baldwin, I think that there are some lectures going on in town that you might be interested in. There is a man here who lectured at a certain place last week and he is coming back again this week and his subject in general, I think, is one that would interest you. So I went to hear you, your talk then. Your subject was almost entirely on occult subjects, I think and the Ethical Society brought you there. In the course of those lectures, I questioned very much whether- I liked Colonel Dinshah well enough, but there were some things I did not like; there are other things-

JUSTICE- When did you get in touch with him? What we are interested in here, I take it, is when did you get in touch with the use of this machine of his?

DINSHAH- When did you get in touch with me about the Spectro-Chrome System?

BALDWIN- Why, that is just what I'm getting at. Now, you were delivering this course of lectures, you had one of the Spectro-Chrome machines of a different type than this in the room and you at the last lecture said something regarding the use of it as a therapeutic measure and another doctor and myself in the audience went up to you and asked you, why you would not- if you would give a course on the Therapeutics of Color in Philadelphia. Your reply was, "Yes, if you can get up a class, I shall be glad to do so." I said, "I will be one of it." The other doctor said, he would be another one and from that you had your first class in Philadelphia of some eighty, I think somewhere along there, people.

DINSHAH- And there were numerous doctors in it?

BALDWIN- There was quite a number of doctors in it.

DINSHAH- Dental surgeons?

JUSTICE- What year was that?

BALDWIN- That was in 1820.

DINSHAH- 1921?

BALDWIN- 1921, yes. Not 1820. I got my centuries mixed.

DINSHAH- 1921, before you discovered the origination of Spectro-Chrome?

BALDWIN- Yes.

DINSHAH- There were dental surgeons in it?

BALDWIN- Yes, sir.

DINSHAH- Surgeons?

BALDWIN- Yes, sir.

DINSHAH-And lay people?

BALDWIN-Yes, sir.

DINSHAH- After you took the work, you took to the practice of Spectro-Chrome Metry, in your own private practice, as well as your hospital work?

BALDWIN- Yes, sir.

DINSHAH- That was not a machine like that? Kindly look at it (indicating). It was not invented at that time, in 1921?

BALDWIN- That machine did not exist at that time.

DINSHAH- When I told one of the classes in which you were present, that is one of the meetings, that I had now perfected a motor-driven machine that would give much better facility for work, who placed the first order for this equipment with me, without seeing it?

BALDWIN- I have the first machine of that kind that was made.

DINSHAH- You have the first machine exactly of that type?

BALDWIN- Yes, sir.

DINSHAH- Was it delivered to you in 1922?

BALDWIN- I couldn't say as to that. About that time.

DINSHAH- About that. If I said you had that machine in your hands since about eight years, seven or eight years, would that be right?

BALDWIN- Yes.

DINSHAH- Did you use that equipment with slide-carrier just like this (indicating)? Kindly examine the glasses and see if those are similar to what you have?

BALDWIN- I should say it was.

DINSHAH- Sealed like that also?

BALDWIN- Yes, sir.

DINSHAH- How many such equipments did you get from the Institute since then?

BALDWIN- Well, I am running eleven every day! And I have several others that I put in homes, where people can not come to me.

DINSHAH- About how many in all, Spectro-Chrome equipments?

BALDWIN- Different kinds of equipment, not of that kind.

DINSHAH- Have you three like that?

BALDWIN- Yes, sir; I have five of them.

DINSHAH- You have five like that?

BALDWIN- Yes, sir.

DINSHAH- Purchased, taken from the Institute at various times, for your work there?

BALDWIN- Yes, sir.

DINSHAH- And you have other Spectro-Chromes. With different arrangement of the work?

BALDWIN- Yes, Colors being the same.

DINSHAH- The Color slides being the same?

JUSTICE- You use eleven every day?

BALDWIN- Yes, sir.

DINSHAH- Using eleven instruments every day?

BALDWIN- Using eleven instruments every day; not all of that type.

DINSHAH- But you have five like that in use?

BALDWIN- I have five like that in use.

DINSHAH- Did you use that in the hospital where you were?

BALDWIN- Not this type.

DINSHAH- No, the other type that you had?

BALDWIN- I did, yes, sir.

DINSHAH- With the same kind of slides?

BALDWIN- Yes, sir.

DINSHAH- Same Color slides?

BALDWIN- Yes, sir.

DINSHAH- Do you remember a case of burns of a girl, Grace Shirlow by name?

BALDWIN- Yes, sir.

DINSHAH- Produce the pictures of the condition of the girl and what you did. (Baldwin produces the pictures.)

DINSHAH- I present to you, please, Doctor- these will have to be separated- this picture. Do you identify the girl that is shown there, as the condition of the girl after she was burnt by fire (showing photogram to witness)?

BALDWIN- Yes, sir.

DINSHAH- How much was she burnt in the front, in that picture as you made?

BALDWIN- About four-fifths of the torso was burnt; that is, the trunk. This represents the middle of the body here (indicating). She was burnt beyond the middle of the body; it went up to the clavicle and under the arm.

JUSTICE- That is the shoulder blade, as we call it?

BALDWIN- No, the clavicle. The shoulder blade is on the back.

DINSHAH- Collar bone?

BALDWIN- Collar bone, and it went from the elbow up clear into the axillary, down to the groin, about four inches on the left leg, back up onto the back and around onto this side (indicating); to make it brief, as near as I can, there was about that much (indicating) of the trunk of the body, the torso, as we call it and up to here (indicating) that was not burned; all through here and on the left side of the back, it was not only the skin that was destroyed but the fascia of the muscle-

DINSHAH- What do you mean by fascia?

BALDWIN- The covering of the muscle, so that the little muscle fibers were exposed.

DINSHAH- Just a minute, please. This is the front of that girl (showing photogram to witness)?

BALDWIN- That is the front.

DINSHAH- This is the back (showing another photogram to witness)?

BALDWIN- Yes, sir.

DINSHAH- Identify those photograms, please. (The referred photograms were marked defendant's exhibits 26 and 27 for identification.)

BALDWIN- May I make one statement, in regard to that picture?

DINSHAH- Yes, please, while I am exhibiting.

BALDWIN- That picture was not taken until two weeks after the burn.

DINSHAH- So really the burn was more severe than that?

BALDWIN- The burn was more severe than that. I had cleared up quite a little in the two weeks.

JUSTICE- Do you want to offer them into evidence, Doctor?

DINSHAH-Yes, I did have them in evidence.

JUSTICE- Go right along with your questions. They can examine it.

DINSHAH- This case was brought to you and it came under your surgical care?

BALDWIN- Yes, sir.

DINSHAH- By looking at that case, from your surgical experience and your knowledge of surgery, did you believe that any method known to medicine and surgery, could have kept that child alive?

BALDWIN- It is generally conceded, that with that much of the body burned, even though the surface only may be involved, can not be saved.

DINSHAH- That is, it was an absolutely hopeless, fatal case?

BALDWIN- It was an absolutely hopeless, fatal case. In fact, I got that about 24 hours after the burn and the surgeon or the doctor who had been called in, went out very legitimately, just simply wrapped it up in gauze and cotton to protect it, as he was quite justified in saying, "There is no use in trying to do anything with this!" In fact, the dressing was so tightly pressed into the raw surface, that it was two weeks before I succeeded in getting it all off, as I would not force it off. I had to wait until the healing process took place underneath and it loosened up, because if you pulled off the dressings, you would pull off new tissues, as well as old.

JUSTICE- You did use this machine or a similar machine, in connection with the treatment of that case?

BALDWIN- I used it entirely. I said to myself, "There is nothing in regular medicine or surgery, that can make that child live. If I can make it live, it has got to be by something else." Spectro-Chrome Metry was the thing I was working with at the time and I said to my assistant, "We will see what Spectro-Chrome will do." That child had absolutely nothing but Color and diet and dressing of sterilized waxed paper all through. We put a sheet of paper and a sheet of cloth and put in a sterilizer; it took out the parrafin, whatever it was made of, out and left just a sterilized, absorbent paper, very thin. You could see the tissues underneath to a certain extent. We had some sterilized coconut oil, which we ran this paper through. It was so light in weight, but letting it go a little beyond the burn, it did not break off, it would stick to the burn. If in a new dressing, there was any place that stuck, that had not loosened up, we go around it and let it stay on. That child's elimination was kept perfect. She had two and three good bowel eliminations, in the course of 24 hours. She was put on a special diet and given all the lemonade, sweetened with brown sugar, that she could have. That was her principle drink. She had all that she wanted. Do you wish me to go on with the treatment?

DINSHAH- What did you use exclusively for building the skin?

BALDWIN- Well, we had to get rid of-

DINSHAH- I mean, what System did you use? Did you use any medicine or surgery, for building the skin?

BALDWIN- I used no surgery at all.

JUSTICE- That is, you just used this treatment you have described, Doctor?

BALDWIN- I used this treatment.

JUSTICE- Just oil and paper to cover, to keep the air from it and application of Color rays?

BALDWIN- That is all, yes. Just for a minute; we did put a garment over. We could not put a bandage on that you know, because it would have given her pain, so we simply laid down one or two thicknesses of gauze on the bed and put her on it and another over and the nurse sewed it up like, sort of, a little kimono, that simply protected her a little bit from the air No bandages were used, because they would have added pain rather than otherwise.

DINSHAH- You know this, you were taught this Spectro-Chrome Therapeutical System chart (indicating)?

BALDWIN- Yes.

DINSHAH- Did you use this to select your [Color] waves?

BALDWIN- Yes.

DINSHAH- Will you kindly tell the honorable court and the jury, what wave you picked out to build the skin?

BALDWIN- We used the turquoise principally to build the skin.

DINSHAH- That is what you were taught?

BALDWIN- Yes, that is what I was taught.

DINSHAH- How is a turquoise produced by that instrument- of what Colors combined?

BALDWIN- Green, and blue added to green.

DINSHAH- And that makes this turquoise Color?

BALDWIN- That makes the turquoise.

DINSHAH- And it is that which built the skin, on this girl, exclusively?

BALDWIN- No; may have built the skin exclusively. We had to use other Colors to stimulate the separation of the sloughs off body and get rid of that- that dead tissue, before you can build new. New epithelium, new skin, will not cover over dead tissue and we had to stimulate that separation by using stimulating Colors.

JUSTICE- Turquoise was produced, you say, green on blue?

BALDWIN- Green and blue, and her general system had to be kept up. We had to pay attention to her heart condition, to keep that up. I used other things than just simply the turquoise but the turquoise was the thing that probably built the skin in the end. There has never been a known case, as far as medicine and surgery goes, that covered as much surface of the body that was burned, that has ever gotten well. A good many surgeons saw the case and the general opinion was that- well, I know one surgeon, been in the war, he had been all over everywhere, says, "Well, we don't try to treat one of those; we give them just a big dose of morphine and push them off to one side."

DINSHAH- You used Spectro-Chrome on this girl exclusively, without any medical or surgical treatment of any kind?

BALDWIN- No; I was criticized for not skin grafting but what could I skin graft there? No place to skin graft.

DINSHAH- You used only the Spectro-Chrome System?

BALDWIN- I used only the Spectro-Chrome System.

DINSHAH- As taught by Dinshah?

BALDWIN- As taught by Dinshah. The first day she was in the hospital, I was out of town and she was nervous and the intern did not know what to do, had to resort to some bromide.

DINSHAH- You did not give it?

BALDWIN- But she had it, whether I gave it or not. The first day, she was left in the intern's care and the first day she was in, I was out of town and the intern gave her either three or five grains of bromide of sodium. With that exception, that child had not one single thing, except her diet and Spectro-Chrome with the oiled paper.

DINSHAH- Who taught that diet system to you?

BALDWIN- You did.

DINSHAH- How long did it take to complete the building of the body of this little girl, Doctor, so that she could wear a garment again?

BALDWIN- About seven months.

DINSHAH- Seven months?

BALDWIN- It would not have taken that long, had the child- had we been able to give the child the care that a private patient with a private Nurse would have had. We were very scarce of nurses, as all hospitals were at that time. She had to take whatever she could get, of whatever nurse had to be on duty.

DINSHAH- Just a minute, please, Doctor. We shall curtail the examination. You see, I want to save the time. Now, do you remember an incident, during this rebuilding of this skin process, where the Health Authorities did something to this girl and something happened?

BALDWIN- Yes. There was a case of diphtheria in the ward and without saying anything to me about it, they knew I did not approve of injections by interns, so they went around and gave every child in the place a dose of antitoxin.

DINSHAH- Did Grace Shirlow get it too?

BALDWIN- Grace Shirlow did.

DINSHAH- Without your knowledge or consent?

BALDWIN- Yes, sir.

DINSHAH- And what happened to her?

BALDWIN- She had run up a high temperature and was very, very much worse in every way.

DINSHAH- What was the temperature in degrees?

BALDWIN- 105 and 106.

DINSHAH- What brought it down to normal?

BALDWIN- Spectro-Chrome.

DINSHAH- Did you use the Blue Color to reduce this temperature?

BALDWIN- I probably ran it down lower than the Blue Color.

DINSHAH- Used Indigo Color also?

BALDWIN- Indigo; yes, sir.

DINSHAH- You used Blue also?

BALDWIN- I used Turquoise, Blue, Indigo and Violet.

DINSHAH- According to the requirement?

BALDWIN- According to the requirement.

DINSHAH- As taught by my system in the Class?

BALDWIN- Yes, sir.

DINSHAH- And that brought it down to normal?

BALDWIN- Yes, sir.

DINSHAH- Will you please identify these two pictures, of the front and back of the girl, as she was when restored by Spectro-Chrome (showing pictures to witness)?

BALDWIN- Yes.

DINSHAH- I offer them as exhibits.

(The photograms referred were received in evidence and marked defendant's exhibits 28 and 29.)

BALDWIN- There is no cheloid there, Judge, at all or any adhesions to the tissues below.

DINSHAH- Was the skin just like an ordinary skin, movable?

BALDWIN- It was perfectly movable.

DINSHAH- It was not merely a scar tissue but a real skin?

BALDWIN- Yes.

DINSHAH- Thank you. Now, since that period, when you started to experiment about and get the evidence in Spectro-Chrome, I am naming certain things here and you may simply answer by "yes" or "no" whether you used it for these disorders, because we do not have to waste time by going into details of medical work. Did you have cases of cataract of the eyes, restored to normal by Spectro-Chrome?

BALDWIN- Yes.

DINSHAH- Glaucoma or hardening of the eyeballs?

BALDWIN- Yes.

DINSHAH- Acute infections affecting the eyes?

BALDWIN- Yes.

DINSHAH- Hemorrhages in the eyes, that is bleeding?

BALDWIN- Yes.

DINSHAH- About the ears- any mastoid trouble, behind the ears?

BALDWIN- Yes.

DINSHAH- Otitis media, meaning inflammation in the middle ear?

BALDWIN- Yes.

DINSHAH- Any tonsils and adenoids?

BALDWIN- Yes.

DINSHAH- Did you have any experience in the hospitals or in cases in treating bronchial or lung troubles?

BALDWIN- Yes, I had some advanced cases of tuberculosis.

DINSHAH- Bronchitis, I mean, bronchitis, inflammation of the bronchial passages?

BALDWIN- Yes, sir.

DINSHAH- Did you get any cases of pleurisy?

BALDWIN- Yes.

DINSHAH- Any advanced cases of tuberculosis, where cavities were formed and proved to be existent by X-rays, in the lungs?

BALDWIN- Yes, sir.

DINSHAH- Did you use the Spectro-Chrome for functional disorders of the heart?

BALDWIN- Yes.

DINSHAH- Now, did you have occasion to use Spectro-Chrome for gastric ulcers?

BALDWIN- Yes.

DINSHAH- That is, ulcers in the stomach?

BALDWIN- Yes.

DINSHAH- Cancerous conditions?

BALDWIN- Yes.

DINSHAH- Piles or hemorrhoids in the rectal region?

BALDWIN- Yes.

DINSHAH- Abscesses and carbuncles on the back, that big or that big (illustrating with fist) about say, two to three inches in diameter?

BALDWIN- I had carbuncles that reached from here to here (indicating) and from the occiput down to the cervical.

DINSHAH- Would that be about that big or about that big (illustrating with fist)?

BALDWIN- Hardly, spread your hand. Large carbuncles on the neck, that very large one here on the neck (indicating); they have them other places.

DINSHAH- You used Spectro-Chrome for that also?

BALDWIN-Yes, sir.

DINSHAH- Suppresion of urine in this burned girl; was that relieved by Spectro-Chrome?

BALDWIN- Yes, sir.

DINSHAH- Did you use this for the correction of opium, morphine and other drug habits?

BALDWIN- Yes, sir.

DINSHAH- Did you use Spectro-Chrome for any cases of paralysis or palsy?

BALDWIN- Yes, sir.

DINSHAH- Did you get under your surgical treatment there with Spectro-Chrome, and cases of asthma?

BALDWIN- Yes, sir.

DINSHAH- Hay fever?

BALDWIN- Yes.

DINSHAH- Common colds?

BALDWIN- Yes.

DINSHAH- Laryngitis?

BALDWIN- Yes.

DINSHAH- All sorts of infections?

BALDWIN- Yes.

DINSHAH- Mouth disorders?

BALDWIN- Yes.

DINSHAH- Rheumatism, lumbago and such other such other infective disorders with rheumatic fevers?

BALDWIN- Yes.

DINSHAH- Did you have any girl's case of gonorrhea?

BALDWIN- Yes.

DINSHAH- What was the age of the girl?

BALDWIN- Eight years old.

DINSHAH- Eight years old with gonorrhea? What did you do for her?

BALDWIN- Spectro-Chrome.

DINSHAH- Did you have a woman's case there, at the time Grace Shirlow was there, who had syphilis?

BALDWIN- Yes.

DINSHAH- When I came to the hospital, to see Grace Shirlow, do you remember showing me the case of a woman, who was burned by radium and X-rays, so that her palate was ulcerated and so on?

BALDWIN- That one with the roof of the mouth gone?

DINSHAH- Yes. Was not one burnt by radium and X-ray?

BALDWIN- The one with the clavicle and whole front of the body and down the arm here. that was an X-ray burn.

DINSHAH- Did you use Spectro-Chrome for that dangerous case also?

BALDWIN- Yes, sir.

DINSHAH- What was the result?

BALDWIN- It finally healed.

DINSHAH- So, in fact, without going into medical details and so on, you have used Spectro-Chrome in very many of these cases and in fact dangerous cases?

BALDWIN- Yes.

DINSHAH- What has been your experience in the use of the System?

BALDWIN- Absolutely satisfactory. They will always need an undertaker. We do not claim that, you know.

DINSHAH- Beg your pardon?

BALDWIN- We will always need the undertaker. We do not claim that we will not, but anything that is in human possibility to be put in a normal shape, it can be done with Spectro-Chrome better than it can with anything else and with many, many cases, it is the only thing that would put the patient in a condition to function.

DINSHAH- You had experience in venereal disorders?

BALDWIN- Yes, sir.

DINSHAH- What was your experience with Spectro-Chrome, in tonating those cases?

BALDWIN- They came out alright.

DINSHAH- Then, in fact, you will correct me if I am wrong, that you are still using Spectro-Chrome, stronger than ever?

BALDWIN- I use practically nothing else.

DINSHAH- But Spectro-Chrome?

BALDWIN- But Spectro-Chrome.

DINSHAH- Now, I shall show to you this chart again-

JUSTICE- That is exhibit 10.

DINSHAH-Your Honor, People's exhibit 10; yes, sir.

JUSTICE- So as to identify the chart.

DINSHAH- Yes, sir. People's exhibit 10.

DINSHAH- This Spectro-Chrome therapeutic system, in your experience and knowledge as a physician, looking to the physiological effects produced by these Color waves, did you find that these effects are actually produced or did you find that the chart is humbug?

BALDWIN- In all general ways, the chart is not a humbug-absolutely.

DINSHAH- What is your experience from the results?

BALDWIN- My experience from the results is, that the chart is correct.

DINSHAH- You were in the class in Philadelphia. Did your interest increase so much, that you wanted to repeat it, for your own knowledge?

BALDWIN- Yes, sir.

DINSHAH- How many classes and courses did you take and pay for in full?

BALDWIN- Five.

DINSHAH- You paid me for all of them?

BALDWIN- I paid you for five in full. I took one course afterwards by your invitation.

DINSHAH- And what was the purpose in repeating the courses?

BALDWIN- That I might get more general knowledge.

DINSHAH- Was it necessary that you repeat them?

BALDWIN- I probably learned a good deal, but I may say, all my good work, was done before I repeated, but I do not think you can ever stop learning. If the doctors stop learning, when they came out of medical College, they would know mighty little; they would be of mighty little good to the community, less than they are as it is.

DINSHAH- Do you know as a physician in your County and State work with other medical Societies, whether your friend doctors are also using now various systems of Color and Light, for healing purposes?

BALDWIN- There is practically no hospital that I know of, that is not using Light, plain Light or some colored Lights, in some way and there are great many of our physicians, who are using Color and Light in their private work. Very few were doing it when Spectro-Chrome was put in evidence.

DINSHAH- Do you remember in Philadelphia, the Jefferson University introducing it recently?

BALDWIN- Well, I know that they do use Light and Color there.

DINSHAH- In Jefferson?

BALDWIN- Yes.

DINSHAH- That is a great University, is it not, don't you know?

BALDWIN- Well, it is one of the best medical colleges in the world.

DINSHAH- Now, Doctor, a little more clarification: in the class work, you heard me playing an organ?

BALDWIN- Yes.

DINSHAH- What was the purpose of that organ, in demonstrating what?

BALDWIN- The similarity between or the connection between sound waves and Color waves, Light waves.

DINSHAH- What is taught by- what is the connection taught, I mean as regards the oscillatory frequencies of sound and so on? Is there any apparatus in the class or is it by word of mouth only?

BALDWIN- There is an organ on which you demonstrate oscillatory frequencies.

DINSHAH- On the organ?

BALDWIN- On the organ.

DINSHAH- The organ is not for mere entertainment, then; it has a purpose of oscillatory frequencies?

BALDWIN- Absolutely.

DINSHAH- How long do I play the organ, just in the beginning to request the Divine Architect of the Universe to help the work? In the beginning of the class work, how long do I invoke the Deity's help, by the organ and a song or hymn? How long does it take?

BALDWIN- Three to five minutes; I should say, never more than five, perhaps not more than three minutes many times.

DINSHAH- Is the work, according to your viewpoint in a medical college, conducted along scientific grounds or merely as just a fake system to get money?

BALDWIN- Absolutely most scientific thing there is in the healing art today.

DINSHAH- You studied other courses in medicine, surgery and other things?

BALDWIN- I have been through the regular mill.

DINSHAH- Is there any course that you really can compare in the science of spectroscopy, with this course?

BALDWIN- Not at all.

DINSHAH- In our work, that is?

BALDWIN- Yes, sir.

DINSHAH- Do I show the relation of chemicals of the human body to the Color waves?

BALDWIN- Yes.

DINSHAH- I offer this People's exhibit 10 again for you to identify here; the chemical chart, as is put there, is step by step experimentally demonstrated with chemical tubes and Spectroscopy; this chart?

BALDWIN- It is.

DINSHAH- And is found to be just exactly as I teach it or is it merely a fluke, to your mind?

BALDWIN- It is an absolute guide.

DINSHAH- I shall show you a few of these charts, whether you learned from me. Is this chart always in my Class Room (indicating and showing to witness)?

BALDWIN- Yes, sir, practically always.

DINSHAH- You remember it? Learning from it?

BALDWIN- Yes, sir.

JUSTICE- There does not seem to be any dispute about these charts, Doctor.

DINSHAH- We shall drop that, Your Honor, I shall save your time, sir. Were you ever to the Spectro-Chrome Institute, at Malaga, New Jersey, the central office of this work?

BALDWIN- Yes.

DINSHAH- Is this the place (showing photogram to witness)?

BALDWIN- I should say it was, yes.

DINSHAH- How many acres are there? How big is that place?

BALDWIN- You have got about 23, about that.

DINSHAH- 23 acres. How many buildings are there?

BALDWIN- Four or five.

DINSHAH- There is an auditorium and research laboratory there?

BALDWIN- Yes, they are together in one building.

DINSHAH- Resident quarters?

BALDWIN- Yes, sir.

DINSHAH- Administration building?

BALDWIN- The administration building and the auditorium is all in one building.

DINSHAH- Printing plant?

BALDWIN- Printing plant.

DINSHAH- So that is not a fly-by-night institution, according to your mind?

BALDWIN- No.

DINSHAH- But a real laboratory for serving humanity?

BALDWIN- It is a real laboratory, sir, serving humanity.

DINSHAH- I shall offer this into evidence.

(The photogram was received in evidence and marked defendant's exhibit 30.)

DINSHAH- You dealt with this Spectro-Chrome Institute for the last 10 years now, nearly?

BALDWIN- Yes, sir.

DINSHAH- In their relations with the public, as you judged from your own experience, how did you find them?

BALDWIN- I have always found them perfectly honest and square, with the intent to do the straight thing.

DINSHAH- Do they fulfill their contracts?

BALDWIN- Certainly.

DINSHAH- Do they fulfill whatever they tell in the classroom, as their word of honor?

BALDWIN- Yes, sir.

DINSHAH- Did you ever have any reason to complain against the Institute?

BALDWIN- I have never issued a complaint.

DINSHAH- Was there any reason to issue one?

BALDWIN- If there had been, I certainly should have put it in.

DINSHAH- Thank you. Please take the witness.

After Dinshah concluded his direct examination of Dr. Baldwin, the Plaintiff was allowed to cross examine her. The cross examination now follows:

HAGERTY- Doctor, isn't the use of waxed paper or paraffin recognized as the standard treatment of burns?

BALDWIN- Yes, but naturally there is no paraffin or wax left in the paper after it has been sterilized.

HAGERTY- But the use of waxed paper or paraffin is recognized as a standard treatment of burns?

BALDWIN- Paraffin is, yes, paraffin is sprayed over the parts very many times, but there was no paraffin or wax left in the paper; it was all taken out by the cloth; there was one layer of cloth and also of paper and put in a sterilizer; there was not a bit of wax left in it.

HAGERTY- You mean, when this girl's picture was taken here, she was treated, instead of following the usual procedure or following the standard treatment of burns, by using wax paper or paraffin that the paper was treated so that the paraffin or wax was taken out of the paper?

BALDWIN- Yes, sir.

HAGERTY- Did you then use an absolutely radical change from what was recognized the standard treatment?

BALDWIN- I had been in the habit of using thin silk for a long time, but silk was most too expensive for an extensive thing like that.

HAGERTY- What I am getting at is, in this particular case that you have spoken of as far as you knew, up to that time, one of these standard- at least one of the standard treatments of burns was the use of waxed paper, then in the treatment of this case, that standard treatment was departed from entirely by taking the wax out of the paper?

BALDWIN- By taking the wax out of the paper; the standard treatment there with the wax was more to spray it on in some way than it was to just use a waxed paper to put on.

HAGERTY- Was the nature of this girl's burn, Doctor, was it primary or- what was the-

BALDWIN- You mean whether it was first, second, or third degree burn?

HAGERTY- Yes.

BALDWIN- It was burn from fire. Her clothes caught afire and it was all the grades in different parts, from the first degree to the third degree burn.

HAGERTY- If too much damage has not been done by a burn and this standard treatment of waxed paper or paraffin, spraying of paraffin is used, it would effect a complete cure, would it not?

BALDWIN- Just state that again.

HAGERTY- If, in case of burn, where the damage was not too extensive, what I mean by that, not too-

BALDWIN- All are the third degree burns, yes. I understand what you mean.

HAGERTY- I do not mean in area, if not damaged too much, this standard treatment of waxed paper or paraffin would effect a complete cure, would it not?

BALDWIN- In some cases it would, yes, but there are other cases that are so damaged that is when we know the paraffin was not taken up by every surgeon by any means.

HAGERTY- And this covering of this girl's body with this paper, which you have described was continued, was it, during the course of her convalescence?

BALDWIN- Yes, sir.

HAGERTY- And she was put on a diet, in other words, to build her system up and so forth?

BALDWIN- To build her system up. In a general way, yes, we looked after the elimination and the building up diet.

HAGERTY- How long after she came inside the hospital, was the Spectro-Chrome used or this Spectro-Chrome started?

BALDWIN- About two hours.

HAGERTY- Two hours after she came into the hospital?

BALDWIN- She still was having the effect of the burn itself, that is, the stinging, burning, so forth, so we put her immediately on Spectro-Chrome to overcome that.

HAGERTY- The cause of death from a burn like that- what is the direct cause of death?

BALDWIN- Well, it is usually a lack of elimination through the skin, the functioning of the skin and the kidneys are very apt to go off.

HAGERTY- It is some kind of a poisoning developed?

BALDWIN- It is some kind of a poisoning developed; there is no way of eliminating the poison; we eliminate a great deal of the poison through the skin and the kidneys and the bowels and the lungs.

JUSTICE- Comes out through this process of perspiration?

BALDWIN- Yes.

HAGERTY- What kind of poisoning do you call that? Is that uremic?

BALDWIN- Well, there is no special name for it, as I know of; it is a toxic condition; depends a good deal upon what was in the- you get a toxic condition from the tissues that are being thrown off; whatever condition the patient may be in, would determine to a great extent what toxin it would throw off.

HAGERTY- So that a person's recovery from a burn, depends a whole lot upon the elimination?

BALDWIN- A whole lot upon the elimination, yes.

HAGERTY- And if the poison which has developed can be eliminated in various ways, through the bowels and so forth, their chances of recovery are so much better?

BALDWIN- Certainly

HAGERTY- How old was this child, this girl?

BALDWIN- Eight years old.

HAGERTY- So that the possibilities are that her physical condition and her process of elimination were in very good condition, were they not?

BALDWIN- Very good, yes. She was not a child that had been properly fed or brought up at all; she was the middle one of seven children, with but enough money to take care of two.

HAGERTY- Are you a member of the American Medical Association?

BALDWIN- Yes, sir.

HAGERTY- And do you know whether this Jefferson Hospital is a chartered university?

BALDWIN- Oh, yes. It is one of the oldest medical Schools in the Country.

JUSTICE- Is that connected with the University of Pennsylvania?

BALDWIN- No, sir, it is a separate institution entirely.

HAGERTY- Have you abandoned the practice of medicine?

BALDWIN- No, I have not abandoned it. I use it if I have to, but I shall not use it as long as I can get Spectro-Chrome; if I was cut out somewhere where I could not get Spectro-Chrome, I would have to go back to the next best thing.

HAGERTY- You apparently have been convinced, through the teachings of the Colonel and other things, that Spectro-Chrome surpasses medicine?

BALDWIN- Only if in a matter of emergency that I would use the old methods of treatment.

HAGERTY- How long have you been in that frame of mind?

BALDWIN- Well, I commenced to use Spectro-Chrome the latter part of 1920 or first of 1921 and it did not take me very long to decide that it was better than anything else I had.

HAGERTY- And then, if I understand your testimony correctly, you are of the opinion too, that Spectro-Chrome will cure anything and everything?

BALDWIN- No, there was not anything on the face of the Earth that will cure anything and everything. We have all of us got to die some time.

HAGERTY- Well, of course, I do not mean that. There is always a time when we are going to die; you are going to die, I suppose. What I mean, Doctor, is that it will cure any of the so-called diseases?

BALDWIN- Any of the so-called diseases, any that is reasonably curable, it will cure and it will cure many things which drugs and general surgery and surgical work will not and surgical work will do better- cases of surgery will do better, if you use Spectro-Chrome in connection with it, than if you use only the old surgical method.

HAGERTY- It will cure dementia praecox, will it?

BALDWIN- Other people have had those cases and cured them. I have not had a case of that brought it.

HAGERTY- Would you cure the dementia praecox then, before you found out that-

BALDWIN- I never had a case of it in my whole practice.

HAGERTY- You never had a case of that in your whole practice?

BALDWIN- No.

HAGERTY- Did you study it?

BALDWIN- Yes.

HAGERTY- It is a mental disease, is it not?

BALDWIN- Yes, we had a general course in mental diseases.

HAGERTY- Was there a cure for it, before Spectro-Chrome could cure it, do you know?

BALDWIN- Well, there was never any definite cure for it; some would use one method and some would use another; good many cases were cured and some cases were not cured.

JUSTICE- It is generally recognized as incurable, is it?

BALDWIN- Permanently incurable.

HAGERTY- That is, as far as the medical profession has been concerned, it was recognized as incurable, either by surgery or by medicine, drugs?

BALDWIN- Yes.

HAGERTY- But you know of cases that have been cured by Spectro-Chrome?

BALDWIN- Not personally.

HAGERTY- I mean, you have not treated them personally, but you have-

BALDWIN- I have heard people say that they have-

DINSHAH- Your Honor, hearsay evidence can not be admitted.

JUSTICE- Well, it is helping you.

DINSHAH- Yes, even then, I am fair to the other party too. We shall stick to the law; your own personal experience.

JUSTICE- I think the Colonel is right.

HAGERTY- It will cure my venereal disease?

BALDWIN- It, in my hands, has cured gonorrhea and syphilis.

HAGERTY- Syphilis?

BALDWIN- Yes, sir.

HAGERTY- As far as the medical profession is concerned, syphilis, when it reaches a certain stage, was generally recognized as incurable, was it not?

BALDWIN- No, not now. We can usually find something in the regular medical work, surgery, that will eventually heal the destructive process.

HAGERTY- It will stop it?

BALDWIN- It will stop it, yes.

HAGERTY- It will stop the disease but it won't cure it?

BALDWIN- Well, you can get it so that the general tests for the disease are negative.

HAGERTY- Will Spectro-Chrome cure tuberculosis?

BALDWIN-Yes, sir.

HAGERTY- And will it cure cancer?

BALDWIN- In many cases of cancer, it will, if there has not been too much destruction of tissue. Spectro-Chrome will cure it, will build up the tissue. If it has to come to operation and there is a great deal of destruction of tissue it will simply make them comfortable for the rest of their lives, but it will make them comfortable so that they can enjoy the rest of their life to a certain extent, without doping them with opiates.

HAGERTY- There are a great many world recognized physicians who are attempting to find a cure for cancer, are there not?

BALDWIN- Yes, it is one of the hard things that the medical world is trying to do and they have not gotten very far with it.

HAGERTY- But Spectro-Chrome will cure it?

BALDWIN- I say Spectro-Chrome with- not an advanced case will cure it, on the surface like the epithelium; I have had a number of those that were cured.

HAGERTY- And the medical world has always been looking for a cure for tuberculosis too, has it not?

BALDWIN- Yes.

HAGERTY- But Spectro-Chrome will cure tuberculosis?

BALDWIN- Do you wish a case cited as-

HAGERTY- No, I do not care about going into specific cases. I am just asking your opinion about Spectro-Chrome. That is what I am getting at.

BALDWIN- It has done it, in cases where there were big festers and small festers, where it had been pronounced advanced cases and was ready for the sanatarium, to go into the advanced wards and I have had patients that had been most of the time for three or four years and had been in the sanatarium part of that time, who came under Spectro-Chrome and there is one case now who is back in the sanatarium now nursing, because she says she feels that people who have had tuberculosis and gotten over it, are the ones who should take care of the tubercular people.

HAGERTY- Do you believe in the use of surgery, any more Doctor?

BALDWIN- In some cases, yes; surgery, constructive surgery, is necessary in certain cases.

HAGERTY- Do you believe in any general theory that Spectro-Chrome can take the place of surgery and leave organs with a person that would- perhaps, cancer be taken out by a surgeon?

BALDWIN- Oh, yes! I have had strangulated hernia that had been taken care of by Spectro-Chrome and no further operation. I have had ordinary hernias. The muscles tone up so, that they needed no operation and no trusses and many of those things; but I actually had people brought to me that were billed for the operating table in a few hours and have been taken out of the hospital and brought to my office with appendicitis; they have been wheeled in and have not had their appendix out. I have had various appendix cases, that have been diagnosed appendicitis and advised to have operation, that have never had any operation.

HAGERTY- Will it cure appendicitis and hernia too?

BALDWIN- Yes.

HAGERTY- Besides the other diseases that you have spoken about?

BALDWIN- Yes, sir.

HAGERTY- When a patient comes to you, you diagnose the case, do you not?

BALDWIN- Well, you know, if you have been using and doing a thing, you can not help using the knowledge that you have gained over years of experience. I am not limited, of course, as the layman is, in connection with Spectro-Chrome.

HAGERTY- Well, that is what I am getting at.

BALDWIN- I could use only- if it was possible for me to eliminate all my previous knowledge I could do practically as good work as I do now, with Spectro-Chrome.

HAGERTY- Well, then, do you recognize Colonel Dinshah's teachings that diagnosis is entirely unnecessary?

BALDWIN- Well, diagnosis from the medical standpoint, yes.

HAGERTY- In other words that you join with him in his teachings, that, for instance, it does not make any difference whether a person is suffering from typhoid fever or scarlet fever or any other fever, that it is all a fever and treated by certain Light?

BALDWIN- Any toxic, any septic condition, is practically the same thing.

HAGERTY- Well, you do not, I suppose, believe in that part of the teaching of Colonel Dinshah, do you?

BALDWIN- Well, I think that we treated- most people treat fevers and things to a great extent in the same way.

HAGERTY- That is, they treat scarlet fever, the same as typhoid fever?

BALDWIN- To a great extent by keeping up the elimination and feeding them properly and all that sort of thing, as any layman knows.

HAGERTY- Do you agree then that it does not make any difference, really whether the person's disease like, say tuberculosis, whether it is in the incipient stage or in the advanced stage?

BALDWIN- Well, of course, you can get results quicker in incipient stage than you can in the advanced stage.

HAGERTY- But as far as the treatment is concerned, it is the same then?

BALDWIN- As far as the treatment is concerned not exactly just the same because an advanced case the cavities fill with pus there are cavities as big as that (indicating) in the apex, 2/3 filled with pus or lots of small cavities through the Lung, that absolutely had been healed entirely.

HAGERTY- With Spectro-Chrome?

BALDWIN- According to X-rays.

HAGERTY- You are not connected with any hospital now, Doctor?

BALDWIN- I am not, at the present time, no.

HAGERTY- How long since?

BALDWIN- Three years.

HAGERTY- You say you have got 10 of these machines working. Where are they working?

BALDWIN- Where are they working?

HAGERTY- Yes.

BALDWIN- Well, my office is 1117 Spruce Street and I have the different treatment rooms fixed up there.

HAGARTY- That is, you have your office with different rooms and a machine in each room?

BALDWIN- Yes or two or three machines; that is, they are similar machines. In good many of the treatment rooms- I have two machines, for two different places of the body at the same time, to save their time and my time too.

HAGARTY- But persons who can not come to your office, you install machines in their home?

BALDWIN- Occasionally. I do not do much outside work; I have not time for outside work, in fact, turn down most of the outside work. It seems necessary to come to my office once or twice a week and if I feel they need oftener treatments, I let them take a machine, to use at their home between times.

HAGERTY- You say it is your opinion and your frank and sincere opinion, after you have told us about all the experience you have in medicine, 41 years of general practice and surgery in hospitals and so forth, that if you did not have that practice and knowledge, that you could obtain the same results with this machine?

BALDWIN- If I used all the instruments and the diagnostic instrument that the Colonel has given, I think I could get practically the same results.

HAGERTY- I do not quite understand when you say "Diagnostic Instrument." I thought there was no diagnosis.

BALDWIN- Well, the medical profession would call them diagnostic instruments. They are given instruments which will tell you whether your one place of the body is too cold and the other too hot; one place of the body is feeble and the other is over-stimulated, whether you have a fever or whether you do not have a fever. In reality, you know your different organs are made up of different chemical elements; your liver has not the same chemical elements as your spleen.

HAGERTY- Then part of it there, anyhow, of this apparatus here, you have certain instruments with which you make some kind of a diagnosis?

BALDWIN- Well, if you call it diagnosis, if you wish; the lay people are taught not to use this term "diagnosis."

JUSTICE- That is, because a rose by any other name-

BALDWIN- By any other name, will be just the same, Judge, exactly.

HAGERTY- In other words, the Colonel, in teaching lay people, wants to see that they protect themselves?

BALDWIN- So that they do not get in wrong with the law.

HAGERTY- Prevents the practice of medicine without a licence?

DINSHAH- I object to that question. Nobody is brought here for any violaticn of the law, Your Honor.

JUSTICE- I take it that she does not know what the Colonel thinks?

DINSHAH- That is the idea.

JUSTICE- So I sustain that objection.

HAGERTY- That is, you say the Colonel teaches his lay patients- I suppose the lay patients are any patients who might come, wish to get interested, is that it?

BALDWIN- Yes. I think, the Colonel, if he saw that somebody was entirely unfitted for the work, he would counsel them to not take the course. I do not think he would ever accept a person in his class that he felt was unfitted to take the work, simply for the hundred dollars or whatever his charge.

HAGERTY- In other words, your opinion of the Colonel is, that if somebody came up and undertook this course and paid him one hundred fifty dollars for it and if he found out that he was an entirely unqualified, why, he would not take the money?

BALDWIN- He would say: "Take your $150 back; you are not fitted for this work."

HAGERTY- For instance, if a man has no more qualifications for a course than say, repairing washing machines, lawnmowers and so forth, you believe that if the Colonel knew that, he would give him his money back and tell him not to take the course?

BALDWIN- There are a good many persons with good common sense, where good common sense goes further than lots of technical knowledge and he may be a man that is doing washing machine repairing and lawnmowers, that would have more common sense to bring into his use, than some college- medical college graduates have.

HAGERTY- I did not mean that in criticizing anybody's education.

BALDWIN- Well, his education is the general education, his general common sense and ability to take things in, whether he has had a technical education or not, seems to me, counts quite a good ways.

HAGERTY- You mean, Doctor, that supposing a person has no knowledge whatever of anatomy or has no knowledge at all of Chemicals or of the Sun's rays, any technical knowledge of that, has never done anything during their life about these, leaving out their education, they may be a person of common sense and that by handling some kind of machine, do you believe that then, that person could come home and take a lecture- a course of lectures- sixty hours- and at the end of sixty hours of lecture, talking as the Colonel does and as you heard him, talking fast about chemistry and chemical elements and all these names, that if he then put in the sixty hours of that time, that that person could then take that apparatus and get results from it?

BALDWIN- I think they could, if they used all the apparatus that he has given for finding out what the trouble is.

HAGERTY- And that the results would be the same, those results could be obtained for persons suffering from dementia praecox or a venereal disease or cancer or tuberculosis or ulcers of the stomach or any of those things?

BALDWIN- If they use the means that is given them and stick strictly to what they would come out with a larger percentage of benefits than the average medical doctor does.

HAGERTY- Oh, then, if I understand you, then, you think that a person under those circumstances, would be better equipped to do this, than the average medical doctor?

BALDWIN- I think he would be better equipped after the one course than the ordinary doctor is, when he or she comes out of medical college. You know mighty little, you know, of the human body, when you come out; you have got a lot of technical work, a lot of technical terms, you can give all the bones of the body and the muscles and all their attachments, but you have not any knowledge of a human being, so to speak and your sympathetic nervous system and your occult system, your real self aside from your physical body, is of more importance than your actual bones and muscles are.

HAGERTY- Well, you mean that the medical Student who has, as I understand it, spent several years of studying the body and anatomy and so forth, that when he comes out and also has to serve an internship in the hospital, does he not, before he is admitted into practice?

BALDWIN- In most of the States, they are obliged to.

HAGERTY- So that, how many years, for instance, in Pennsylvania does a young man have to study and then serve an internship and so forth, before he is admitted to practice?

BALDWIN- Well, it is pretty well towards six years before he will get into practice.

HAGERTY- Well, I thought six or seven years here?

BALDWIN- About that time.

HAGERTY- But you believe that the average person who would go and attend one of Colonel Dinshah's course of lectures of 60 hours and graduate and get one of these diplomas, would be better fitted, better equipped to get results than the medical student who has gone through these courses and internship?

BALDWIN- A medical student nowadays, when he comes out of college, depends almost 95% for his ability to do anything, because of the laboratories with which he is associated; everything is sent to the laboratory; medical students are not taught to make outside diagnosis anymore; they really have to depend upon a laboratory report, for practically everything that they do.

HAGERTY- Well, that is in an effort to get the medical profession to make-

BALDWIN- to complicate things.

HAGERTY- Make the diagnosis more certain?

BALDWIN- Well, I suppose it does. It complicates matters very much.

HAGERTY- But in this Spectro-Chrome, diagnosis, it is not necessary, is it?

BALDWIN- Not what- we do not call it diagnosis. You are going to find out whether the person is below par or above par, whether he is on the fever side or the cold side and that is all that medicine does.

HAGERTY- Did Colonel Dinshah, in the course of his teachings, at the various times you have been there, did he tell you that the machine itself diagnoses the case?

BALDWIN- No, sir. That machine does not diagnose anything.

HAGERTY- Well, from what I understand, Doctor, from you-

BALDWIN- Does not tell you anything, as to what to do either; the machine does not.

HAGERTY- I understand, from the way you testified here, you have very definitely turned your back on medicine?

BALDWIN- I have. I would close my office tonight never to see another sick person, unless it was an emergency, if I had to go back to old style medicine and give up Spectro-Chrome. Now, that is just honest- that just represents my belief in Spectro-Chrome.

HAGERTY- Well, that is what I mean. So that you have been completely sold Spectro-Chrome.

BALDWIN-I am completely sold on Spectro-Chrome, and I gave no case in which I had not personally had experience.

HAGERTY- That is all.

As soon as prosecutor Leo Hagerty finished his cross examination, it was Dinshah's turn to try to untangle the confusion created by the cross examination.

DINSHAH- Please, just a little clarification of the points involved, Dr. Baldwin, so as not to leave anything. You spoke about the sympathetic nervous system and so on. I shall show you a chart issued by the Institute, People's exhibit #11. Do you recognize this so-called complicated chart, with foreign words, so forth and so on?

BALDWIN- I do, yes.

DINSHAH- Is this a part of the course?

BALDWIN- Yes.

DINSHAH- What kind of part does it take in this work?

BALDWIN- Well, it goes into the part where the sympathetic nervous system is involved.

DINSHAH- Is the sympathetic nervous system one of the great things that regulates the functions of the human body?

BALDWIN- The sympathetic nervous system regulates all of the automatic functions of the body.

DINSHAH- That is what is known as the autonomous nervous system?

BALDWIN- Yes, your heart keeps on beating, you keep on breathing, your nutrition goes on, all of things go on through the action of the sympathetic nervous system.

DINSHAH- Is this work shown by me, directly stated in the class, by my own self to the students, exemplifying that term just as demonstrated?

BALDWIN- Yes.

DINSHAH- It is.

BALDWIN- Yes.

DINSHAH- Did you ever find any fault in practical work, in your own clinical work, when you applied this work?

BALDWIN- I have not.

DINSHAH- You use it every day in your work?

BALDWIN- I use it everyday; that is, certain parts of it; I do not go into all of this Sanskrit.

DINSHAH- But the American phraseology is beneath to explain it?

BALDWIN- The American phraseology I go into.

DINSHAH- This is a genuine science there?

BALDWIN- A genuine science.

DINSHAH- And you apply it in your daily work?

BALDWIN- I do.

DINSHAH- Now, there is some confusion about this constructive surgery and destructive surgery. I want to qualify that. Does Spectro-Chrome Institute, through my mouth, ever teach that surgery as applied to the human body to build up a broken Bone or anything, is useless?

BALDWIN- No. You have always said that outside of constructive surgery-

DINSHAH- When the Institute says, "No surgery," it simply means "no destructive surgery"?

BALDWIN- No destructive surgery.

DINSHAH- That is, the human body is like a machine; if a part of the machine inside can be saved, save it by Spectro-Chrome if you can, but do not let it be cut off?

BALDWIN- Unless you cannot save it.

DINSHAH- That means, then, to clear the situation in ordinary language, if a woman is sick from any disorder, according to our system, in 60 hours anyone ought to be able to tonate and give service, if we find that part out of equilibrium, that we have the means of repairing that damage and save that part from being taken out?

BALDWIN- In the large proportion of cases, yes.

DINSHAH- And did you do that with Spectro-Chrome?

BALDWIN- I have.

DINSHAH- In constructive surgery then, Spectro-Chrome leads over any other system?

BALDWIN- In constructive surgery, yes and in all other surgery, it will do better, you will get better results if you use Spectro-Chrome in connection with your other surgery, than you will if you trust to your surgery.

DINSHAH- Supposing you had a broken bone- somebody comes with the femur broken or any part- any bone broken and after the surgeon has performed the mechanical work of putting the bones together, what is the idea of Spectro-Chrome?

BALDWIN- In tonating and setting into equilibrium those disorders there. In the first place, you can get a general systemic condition; in another, you can get better nutrition and elimination and all of that will be good and that will help to build the bone, help to nourish the whole body; you have got to pay attention to the whole body. Then, in many times, in broken bones, Nature has not sufficient power to throw out callus and there callus is similar to mending tissue that is thrown out between the ends of the broken bones and in thick Bones, it runs up in, we get a bone callus or get an intermediate callus, a callus that holds it; many times there is not vitality enough to any of that callus thrown out. If we use Spectro-Chrome on that, we will produce the necessary stimulation and the callus will be thrown out. In other condition, there is an excess of callus, which occasions means a deformity.

DINSHAH- Now, Doctor, in this case where it is compulsory, you have to take on the operating table, for instance, a foot that is reduced to a pulp by an automobile truck going on it, which can not be set right, when you must perform a compulsory surgical operation to remove it, you have found Spectro-Chrome even in those cases, useful during the process, when you gave gas for an anesthesia?

BALDWIN- Well, Spectro-Chrome before anesthesia, you mean?

DINSHAH- Yes.

BALDWIN- It makes the anesthetic very much more quietly taken, if you can give the proper Spectro-Chrome, before you send the patient to the operating table, they will take the anesthesia much more quietly and they will recover from it with much less unpleasantness in the way of nausea and vomiting and so forth.

DINSHAH- About this diagnosis which has been put in by the learned counselor, I want to ask you one question: Is medical diagnosis 100% correct?

BALDWIN- It is not claimed to be 100%.

DINSHAH- What is the correct percentage?

262 J. EUGENE WILSON

BALDWIN- The percentage is about from 50 to 52%.

DINSHAH- 52% correct?

BALDWIN- Yes.

DINSHAH- That means that if a person simply adheres to medical and surgical diagnosis, 48% of the people would be ripped open for something they did not have for which to be ripped open?

BALDWIN- I am afraid that I will have to admit that. I am sorry.

DINSHAH- And in Spectro-Chrome, while it does not deal with differential diagnostic names of disorders, is there any chance a person putting the Spectro-Chrome wrongly and damaging the system?

BALDWIN- No, sir.

DINSHAH- Therefore, what is your opinion of Spectro-Chrome, from the standpoint of safety to the public?

BALDWIN- Absolutely. I think I might say, absolutely you can do no real harm with Spectro-Chrome.

DINSHAH- There was a medical gentleman here, who spoke about some Lights, which if put on the eye for an hour would burn it. If that Spectro-Chrome thousand-watt bulb that is there, be put with that Indigo color slide, made by violet and blue together and the eye be put right into the focus of that for an hour, what effect would happen?

BALDWIN- There would be no harm done.

DINSHAH- Can any harm be done to the delicate eye by Spectro-Chrome?

BALDWIN- No, I should say not, from the number of cases I have used it in, directly.

DINSHAH- You had six of those eye cases?

BALDWIN- Of those cases- case came in when the trouble was with the eye, swollen; absolutely used Indigo.

DINSHAH- Something has been said by you about people diagnosis and "diagnostic machine". You do not see a diagnostic machine on exhibit, on the floor there with this instrument?

BALDWIN- It is not here.

DINSHAH- You have one of my so-called "Finding Machine" or Itisometer?

BALDWIN- Yes, sir.

DINSHAH- Is this the chart of that, exhibit number, complaint's #8?

BALDWIN- Yes, sir.

DINSHAH- You use this chart daily in your work?

BALDWIN- Yes, sir.

DINSHAH- And by means of that machine and this chart, what do you determine without using your head altogether, medically, diagnostically or in any manner, what does that machine do for you with the equipment?

BALDWIN- It only tells me what to do for the patient.

DINSHAH- That means, that that is entirely in the machine made by me, which is not on exhibit here, for which this chart is given and taught in the class to use that equipment?

BALDWIN- Yes.

DINSHAH- And if I tell you that that machine is made for those, who do not want to use their head even with that equipment- that is my head in that machine! Is that right?

BALDWIN- That is quite right.

DINSHAH- And the name of that machine is the Itisometer?

BALDWIN- Yes, sir.

DINSHAH- It does not do any diagnostic work according to medicine or surgery?

BALDWIN- No.

DINSHAH- That has only to do with that equipment and Color slides?

BALDWIN- Yes, sir.

DINSHAH- Only that?

BALDWIN- Only that.

DINSHAH- Is it an absolute necessity that that machine should be used?

BALDWIN- To do good work, I should say it is, particularly with the layman. I think that every layman doing work with Color, should use it.

DINSHAH- But a man who is not able to spend so much money and does not want to go and serve to that extent, with that equipment and the 60 hours' knowledge gained in the class, is he able to serve the public with safety?

BALDWIN- Yes, with safety. Under those circumstances, I would say he had better confine himself to his own family, though.

DINSHAH- All right. No questions, Your Honor.

Since the Redirect examination was completed, Prosecutor Hagerty was allowed to Recross Examine Dr. Kate Baldwin.

HAGERTY- What kind of machine is this "Finding Machine," Dr. Baldwin?

BALDWIN- This? That machine (indicating)?

HAGERTY- Yes, the Finding Machine that is?

BALDWIN- Why, it is a machine that is made by Colonel Dinshah, a very delicate, accurate machine which shows you the amount of deviation from the normal that there is.

HAGERTY- So that then, the person really does not have to be qualified in your method, if he has got that?

BALDWIN- If he has got that machine and will follow it, in 99 cases out of 100, he will do good.

HAGERTY- So that if a person has this- what do you call it? Itisometer?

BALDWIN- Itisometer.

HAGERTY- And will apply the Itisometer, the Itisometer will tell him what is-

BALDWIN- What the color should be.

HAGERTY- What is wrong with the person and what the Colors will be to use?

BALDWIN- Yes.

HAGERTY- So that it is really an automatic process, then?

BALDWIN- It is an automatic process; I must say it is automatic; it would be as good a term as any.

The prosecutor was getting into a deeper hole each time he tried to crack through the surgeon's testimony; so he sat down and the Defendant entered into re-redirect examination of the witness.

DINSHAH- That machine is a patented machine, is it not?

BALDWIN- Yes.

DINSHAH- Here is the patent (indicating). Your Honor can take judicial notice of it.

JUSTICE- Of which machine is this?

DINSHAH- The Itisometer. (To witness) Is this the dial of the machine that you are using? The main dial and the auriculator and other parts? I do not want to go into the issues. Is this part of it?

BALDWIN- That is the diagram.

DINSHAH- And does this represent the inside of it, as you saw it in the class room many times or in the laboratory?

BALDWIN- I have never seen the inside of the machine.

DINSHAH- But is this the dial system?

BALDWIN- Yes.

DINSHAH- And it is an electric thermometer in fact, showing which organ is affected?

BALDWIN- That is just about it.

DINSHAH- And in the class I showed that this instrument is sensitive to 1/40th of a degree Fahrenheit, for detecting difference in the circulation and so on? Is that right?

BALDWIN- Yes.

DINSHAH- I offer that patent, #1,724,469, granted by the United States government, August 13, 1929, in exhibit.

(The patent referred was received in evidence and marked defendant's exhibit 31.)

DINSHAH- You use this in your daily practice to avoid using any scientific diagnosis?

BALDWIN- It is so much more exact than anything else, that it is wise to use it

DINSHAH- That is all.

But that was not all. The prosecutor believed he could still tackle the learned surgeon and get from her some point that would help The People of the State of New York. So, he started the grinding mill.

HAGERTY- Did you ever hear of Palmer's machine in chiropractic?

BALDWIN- I know of it. I have never used it. I have seen it demonstrated.

HAGERTY- Is there any difference between them?

BALDWIN- Oh, yes, very great difference between them.

HAGERTY- Between it and Palmer's machine in chiropractic.

DINSHAH- She says she has not seen it.

BALDWIN- I beg your pardon. I have seen it. I said I have never used it.

HAGERTY- It is not in any way similar to the Itisometer?

BALDWIN- I don't know. There may be some similarity somewhere about it. I have not gone into the technicalities of that machine to the extent of saying that there was no similarity.

The prosecutor sat down and more examination commenced from the defendant.

DINSHAH- Dr. Palmer's machine and the Palmer system have nothing to do with Color waves?

BALDWIN- No.

DINSHAH- It is only chiropractic?

BALDWIN- It is only chiropractic.

DINSHAH- Our system has nothing to do with chiropractic in any manner?

BALDWIN- Not at all.

DINSHAH- We use no manipulation?

BALDWIN- No.

DINSHAH- No drugs?

BALDWIN- No.

DINSHAH- No differential diagnosis or surgery in our work?

BALDWIN- No, sir.

DINSHAH- No questions.

The defendant then requested to call for Howard Page.

JUSTICE- Is he a doctor?

DINSHAH- He is a man who was given service by Spectro-Chrome Metry. Do you want me to get only medical people on it?

JUSTICE- I think that is the only one that is competent. So many other factors enter into it. You can see my reason.

DINSHAH- I see your reasons. We shall save time.

JUSTICE- The doctors are competent witnesses.

DINSHAH- Will not my lay graduates also be competent witnesses, from the standpoint of Spectro-Chrome?

JUSTICE- I'm afraid not, Doctor.

DINSHAH- Of the Spectro-Chrome?

JUSTICE- No; I am afraid not.

The defendant bowed to the opinion of the court, and Dr. Kate W. Baldwin left the stand. Her testimony stayed unshaken.

If you are interested in more information, you may contact the Dinshah Health Society, P.O. Box 707, Dept. 3, Malaga, NJ 08328.

Chapter Eighteen

Royal Rife

In my studies on health, I came into contact with information about Rife which made me interested in answering an advertisement about it. When I received and read their response, I decided immediately that I wanted to purchase their "Rife Instrument." I paid $2,195 to buy it.

They state that "Bio Electronic Frequency has been used to improve health since 1934. People worldwide are conducting their own experiments with serious health problems such as Cancer, Diabetes, Arthritis, Headaches, Infections, Pain, and many other conditions. Reports of success with Rife frequency are amazing."

RESULTS OF RIFE TREATMENTS

The testimonials for this machine are great. One lady stated that she has used this machine for treating her cancer of the breast when the cancer pain was so severe that she could not stand to touch her breast to wash it or even let water run over it. She had gone blind in one eye and had a very bad cough that wouldn't go away. She decided that she had nothing to lose, so she bought a Rife machine and after using it for one month, the severe pain left her. Then, she said, for the next several months very strange things happened to her. THE SIGHT

RETURNED TO HER BLIND EYE AND HER COUGH WENT AWAY! Finally, after 6 months, she was absolutely positive she did not have cancer, so she had blood tests taken and they came back negative. Her recovery was complete. (Note by author: There is a blood test called AMAS which has been determined to be 99% accurate in diagnosing cancer, although it doesn't tell you which part of your body has cancer.)

In another instance, a young man caught Mono from his girlfriend, and states he got so sick he wished he were dead. He started using the machine every day, and after two weeks he felt great and states that the Mono was gone. Then he got rid of his girlfriend because she wouldn't use the machine.

One lady said that she took drugs for chronic sinus infection which she has had most of her life. A friend of hers used the machine to get rid of his Gout, so she decided to try it. After using it a couple of times, her sinuses felt great, so she bought her own machine. Now her mother uses her machine for her cancer.

Another lady said for thirty years she had lived out of her medicine cabinet. "I constantly had migraine headaches and other allergy problems." A friend asked her if she wanted to try the Rife Frequency machine but she declined, because she is skeptical about new things. (Note by author: This machine is not exactly new, as Rife's machine was being used in 1934 to help cure cancer.) Finally, she felt that she was coming down with a cold and decided to give it a try. To her surprise, she felt great the next morning and had no sign of a cold. She finally bought her own machine and never gets headaches or allergies anymore and says she never felt better.

One man had a very severe toothache for two weeks. Unfortunately, all of the antibiotics the doctor gave him didn't help. He finally asked his neighbor if he could use that gadget he always talks about. He sat at his neighbor's kitchen table running this thing on about a dozen channels. When he finally got up to leave, he realized that his toothache was gone.

A GREAT DISCOVERY

The scientist Royal Raymond Rife discovered that the unique electronic "signature" of each specific disease can be modified to eliminate nearly every affliction known to man rapidly and harmlessly. The medical doctor who originally confirmed part or all of this discovery included E.C. Rosenow, Sr. (Chief of Bacteriology, 32 years at Mayo Clinic), Irene Diller, (Inst. of Cancer Research, Philadelphia, PA), Virginia Livingston (NJ & San Diego Clinics), and numerous dignitaries from numerous countries such as France, Germany, Canada, Italy, Japan, Quebec, etc.

The University of Southern California sponsored a Special Medical Research team years ago, to evaluate the electronic therapy of Rife's on the terminally ill. An initial success rate of 87.5% was recorded. After Rife developed some improvement on the treatments, EVERY PATIENT, all 16 in the study, had recovered after 130 days without side effects of any kind.

SICK PEOPLE HAVE VERY POOR IMMUNE SYSTEMS

Other medical treatments were either biological or chemical in nature and depended on the body's own immune system to heal the sick. In reality, a sick person has a very poor immune system or one that is temporarily losing the battle. Rife's treatments were based upon a mechanical application of frequency to the body. Rife's discoveries assisted the burden of healing and once this was done, the only problem was to remove the dead disease organisms from the system of the body. Rife discovered that ANY disease can be eliminated with frequencies based on its individual electromagnetic signature.

Rife had a very superb microscope and with it he became the first human being to actually see a living virus in color. His microscope had 5,682 parts and millionaires like Henry Timken (owner of Timken Bearings) financed his work. After nearly 20,000 unsuccessful attempts, Rife finally isolated and identified the human cancer virus AND NAMED IT "Cryptocides Primordiales." He inoculated 400 lab animals with this virus, created 400 tumors, and them eliminated them. He did likewise with many other diseases.

Just as the resonant frequency which shatters a wine glass can only shatter that type of glass, so Rife's frequencies destroy only disease organisms with the same exact pattern of oscillation.

One good thing about Rife's treatments is that there are NO SIDE EFFECTS and they apparently work. Unfortunately, they can only be used for experimental purposes, since the FDA approval would cost 250 million dollars and has not been paid. Fortunately, we all are allowed to purchase such an instrument to be used for investigative purposes.

MY EXPERIENCE WITH RIFE'S MACHINE

The size of the instrument is only 6.5x6.7 inches high by 2.8 inches deep. Biosolutions only weighs about one pound. (Note: the name on the machine is "Bio Solutions." With your order, you receive an operating manual as well as some auto codes. There are 472 auto codes in the memory of Bio Solutions. You may select an auto code instead of trying to program your own channels.

KILL THE VIRUSES BY SHOCKING THEM TO DEATH

It doesn't take much of a shock to kill the parasites in our bodies. They have no resistance to the shocks we are able to give them which we can't even feel. When you use the parasite eliminator of Dr. Clark, you will never feel the shock, but Rife's Frequency is the exception. Although, most of the time, I don't feel any shock using his machine, occasionally I will get a little shock, but it is never harsh. I used the auto code #193 for cancer, which lasts for 33 minutes and has 11 channels. Each channel lasts 3 minutes.

One requirement was that I should drink a lot of water first thing in the morning and right before taking a treatment. This was to help me to get rid of the billions of viruses that would be killed from the shock. Fortunately, you are able to regulate the shock you will receive. Sometimes it seems non-existent and sometimes it seems severe. Since you are only dealing with 9 volts of electricity, it isn't dangerous normally. If you are a heart patient or use a pacemaker, it is probably dangerous. I soon learned to set the white line of the intensity knob at the 11 o'clock position. This enabled me to receive a small shock sometimes but it was never uncomfortable. I wanted to make sure that it was enough of a shock to kill the parasites.

If you have cancer, you may want to try these same treatments to get rid of your cancer. Most assuredly, you will improve your chances if you take the CoQ10 wafers or CoQ10 Gel, plus the L-Carnitine and the other vitamins, minerals and amino acids I recommended.

If you wish to buy a Rife, you may order it. The cost is normally $2,495, but can be found as little as $1,995. Notice: This information is presented for educational purposes only and is not intended to be construed as medical advice, nor is it intended to lead anyone away from a qualified doctor. We urge you to be supervised by health practitioners knowledgeable in treating your particular condition. This instrument is sold only for authorized uses. We do not dispense medical advice, nor do we prescribe remedies or assume any responsibility for those who treat themselves. By ordering this, or any other instrument mentioned in this book, you understand and agree to these conditions. Order from The Royal Library, 2200 King's Hwy, Dept. 7, Port Charlotte, FL 33980.

Chapter Nineteen

Some Ideas You May Have Missed

Insulin Induced Hypoglycemia (IHT) Note: This is a condensation of an article published in Alternative Medicine: The Voice of Health, Burton Goldberg Group, Jan. 2000, page 34f, phone 1-800-333-HEAL.

Insulin was discovered in 1921, and in 1928 Dr. Manfred Sake was using it to treat psychotic symptoms of morphine addicts. Then in 1957, Dr. Surgis Koroljow of New Jersey used IHT to treat two terminally ill patients for severe depression. In one case, the woman was diagnosed with cervical cancer with metastases to the surrounding structures and lymph glands. After being treated for ten weeks, her cancer was in full remission and she was still well after two years. In another case, the female was diagnosed with metastatic melanoma scattered throughout her body. After 15 weeks of IHT, all traces of cancer were gone. According to his widow, Dr. Korgoljow stopped treating cancer patients because of threats from New Jersey officials and oncologists. IHT was reinvestigated by Wayne Martin in 1998 after he learned of Dr. Korgoljow's works. Mother Teresa's physician is using this treatment on cancer patients at the BioPulse medical clinic in Tijuana, Mexico. No one is absolutely certain as to how IHT can cause cancer cell death, but there are numerous theories. When a patient is given IHT treatments, insulin is injected into the body until blood sugar levels become very low. When this happens, oxygen begins to pool in the blood, because without sugar, it can't enter the cells to produce energy. Cancer cells are anaerobic, and can't survive with high oxygen or with a high pH. The insulin induces sleep and the patient is slowly brought back to consciousness with IV glucose. The patient usually wakes up mentally refreshed, hungry and pain free. These are all good signs for cancer patients. At Bio Pulse, the normal number of treatments is up to 35 over an eight-week period. Since cancer is systemic, simply killing the cancer is insufficient as this is not a cure. The patient's immune system must be greatly strengthened, so that the patient can leave with a good plan for living as a cancer survivor. They detoxify the patient, and give him nutritional support, enzymes, chelation therapy, and the necessary education for good health.

I recently read where Roy Barnes, former governor of Georgia, had decided to use about a billion dollars of money recovered from the tobacco manufacturers to discover an effective cancer treatment. I wondered at the first instance when I learned of this why he didn't use about one half or all of this money to learn about all of the cancer cures that have been discovered, and to improve on them. Wouldn't this make more sense than starting from scratch? Starting from scratch makes about as much sense as the fellow who is in the jungle who wants to use his machette to make his own path rather than use one that has already been made.

Prostate cancer is the number one cancer killer of men and breast cancer is the number one killer of women. The number of men killed by prostate cancer is very comparable to the number of women killed by breast cancer, yet nearly $350 million was spent by the National Cancer Institute on breast cancer research whereas only about $90 million was spent by them on prostate cancer research. Unfortunately, the money being spent on cancer research would probably be sufficient if only they would research some of the treatments already discovered.

NEW MIRACLE PROSTATE CANCER TREATMENT

According to a story written by Dr. William C. Douglas in Second Opinion, February 2001, there is a new miracle prostate cancer treatment that is being used in the U.S. and Europe. This treatment may prove to be very beneficial for treating many other types of cancer as well.

We've all heard of hypothermia, which is the condition where your body temperature falls tremendously, and unless you are treated promptly, you may freeze to death. Hyperthermia is the exact opposite. Hyperthermia has achieved a 90% remission rate in Stage I and Stage II Breast and Prostate Cancer.

There are two types of hyperthermia treatments. They are: microwave treatment and radio-wave treatment. The microwave uses microwaves and the radio-wave used radio waves. Of the two, the radio-wave treatment is much more successful than the microwave. In prostate cancer patients, the microwaves cause agonizing urethral pain and burns both cancerous and non-cancerous tissue alike. This has caused most doctors to abandon this form of treatment altogether. The radio wave treatment does not cause urethral pain, so this is the preferred method of treatment.

"The radio wave treatment can heat the cancer two ways: locally, which hits only the affected region, and the whole body. Both types require heating the body to a temperature of 107-111 degrees Fahrenheit. With local treatment, the heat is directed straight at the cancer by passing electromagnetic waves from a transmitter through the patient to a receiving plate. Cancer tissue is more dense than normal tissue and radio waves are more readily absorbed by denser tissue, so the heat is concentrated in the tumor, killing it."

When the cancer of the prostate is discovered, it has normally spread so the whole body treatment is used. Early diagnoses of prostate cancer is nearly impossible, so it has usually spread when it is discovered. Sometimes a doctor will use both local and whole body treatment.

High temperatures kill cancer. When your body is heated, this breaks down glucose into lactic acid, causing your body to enter an acidic state, which is called acidosis. This causes the oxygen supply to decrease tremendously, and since cancer requires some oxygen to survive, the acidosis suffocates the cancer cells.

Low oxygen and high acidity causes a breakdown of the vessels that supply blood to the cancer. We know that our cancer cells have an infrastructure of blood vessels, and any breakdown prevents these cells from dispensing heat, which is also fatal to the cancer.

Unfortunately, most of the U.S. doctors who use this form of treatment are using the microwave form of hyperthermia. Dr. Douglas doesn't recommend this type of treatment for cancer. To get the radio-wave treatment, you may have to go to Europe. This has been approved by the FDA, but U.S. doctors have been slow to change this treatment.

Another good thing about the radio wave treatment is that it damages the membranes, proteins, and enzymes of cancer cells, which makes them much more vulnerable to anti-cancer treatments. In effect, this will make any treatment you may use much more effective.

Dr. Douglas advises: "If you have prostate cancer, do not submit to surgery, but instead contact the North American Hyperthermia Society at 630-571-2904 or . If they can't help you find a doctor using radio-wave hyperthermia, contact the European Society for Hyperthermic Oncology (ESHO). You may contact Dr. Friedrich Douwes directly at the Klinik St. Georg. His mailing address is: Rosenheimer Str. 6-8, 83043 Bad Aibling, Germany. Telephone 49-8061-398-0.

If you don't take care of your prostate, the cancer may return. I suggest that all male adults take the following each day: Saw Palmetto, Pygeum, and Zinc. You can buy the Saw Palmetto and Pygeum in one capsule and normally you should take 30 mg of Zinc each day, but if you have cancer of the prostate, you may want to take 50 mg for a short while. I have taken Saw Palmetto, Pygeum, and Zinc for many years and have never had any prostate problems.

If you wish to subscribe to "Second Opinion", it costs $49 per year and you receive the written material once a month. Write to Second Opinion Publishing, Inc., 7100 Peachtree Dunwoody Rd., Suite 100, Dept. 7, Atlanta, GA 30328. I just learned that Dr. William Campbell Douglas has turned this over to Dr. Robert J. Rowen, M.D., who writes some excellent articles and comes highly recommended.

NEW HOPE FOR COLON CANCER

In the Winter/Spring 2000 edition of the International Association of Cancer Victors and Friends, they indicate that "Cytotoxic chemotherapy is a disaster where colorectal cancer is concerned. In the USA this year, we are going to have 52,000 deaths from colorectal cancer AND NEARLY EVERY ONE IS GOING TO BE A CHEMOTHERAPY FAILURE."

In the April 27, 1974 issue of The Lancet, a British publication, there was an article "Beware of the Ox." Colon cancer is proportional to beef consumption worldwide. The editor claims there is no population with a low level of beef in diet and a high level of colon cancer. Vegetarians are either free entirely of colon cancer or virtually free thereof. If we all will avoid red meat entirely, we can probably avoid colon cancer likewise. Scotland has the highest beef consumption worldwide and they also have the highest death rate from colon cancer.

VITAMIN D CONNECTION

In a study called the Garland study, the first Garland report in the Lancet indicates that there is a vitamin D connection to cancer. They studied the workers of the Hawthorne Works of the Western Electric Co. in Chicago. They found that the 20% of the men with the highest vitamin D level in their blood were having 14.2% per 1000 colon cancers. The 20% of the men with the lowest amount of vitamin D in their blood had 38.9% per 1000 colon cancers. Another study found that the 20% of the population with the lowest amount of vitamin D in their blood were at an 80% greater risk of colon cancer as compared to the 20% of those with the highest level of vitamin D in their blood. These studies were made in a community where large numbers of those tested ate lots of beef. From this we learn as follows: IF YOU DON'T WANT TO GET COLON CANCER, AVOID EATING ANY RED MEAT AND TAKE 5,000 I.U. OF VITAMIN D PER DAY. Until about 15 years ago, the treatment was only to operate. The survival rate for 5 years then was only about 50%. Then 15 years later, the treatment was surgery plus chemotherapy for one year. This only increased the 5 year rate from 50% to 55%. This increase is so small, that I believe that the patient should be told about it and allowed to decide if he or she wants to undergo the horrible treatment of chemotherapy. (Idea: If chemotherapy is administered the right way, the results have been much better.) If all colorectal patients were given Cimetidine for 7 days before cancer therapy to one year after surgery, death from colorectal cancer could be reduced from 52,000 per year to less than 5,000 per year. This is primarily for patients who eat beef.

ORAL UREA FOR LIVER CANCER

In 1985, virtually every liver cancer patient was given chemotherapy. Patient after patient ended up learning that the chemotherapy had failed and that they soon died. Remember also that chemotherapy destroys your immune system even though what you really need is to strengthen your immune system and keep it strong. If you are interested in contacting and joining the International Association of Cancer Victors and Friends, you may contact them at their Northern California office as follows: Grace Moore, RN, President, 5336 Harwood Rd., Dept. 7, San Jose, CA 95124. Their phone number is: 408-448-4094. I highly recommend them.

RAW THYROID,
RAW THYMUS, ETC.

One day I met a lady who came by my office and she was a member of the National Health Federation. When I learned that this was a great organization where I could learn more about health, I decided to join it. I had already learned that it believed in freedom of choice for us. They believe we should not be compelled to take drugs or any treatment, unless we choose to do so, for any ailment or sickness.

She told me that she had a health problem and wasn't able to handle it herself, so she went to a medical doctor. The doctor made his examination and informed her that she had breast cancer, and told her he would put her on chemotherapy. She said, "Like hell you will." She then agreed to take radiation.

After she had taken radiation for several months and got no better, she decided to visit another doctor. She had him examine her for cancer, and he told her that she was cancer free. He learned that she had been taking radiation, so he told her that her immune system was almost destroyed and that she never had cancer. He sent her to a physician who could determine how much immune system she had left, if any. Sure enough, she scored a 15 out of a possible 100, as I recall. He told her that she could rebuild her immune system by taking the following drops: Raw thyroid, raw thymus, raw multiple glandular, and raw multiple organ. She may have taken other things, but she rebuilt her immune system so that she scored a 55. Every now and then, she would have a setback, and would regress with some kind of health problem. Her score would then drop back down to as low as 30, and then she would have to rebuild it.

She lived alone, and one day she suffered a stroke while she was at home. She fell to the floor and when she recovered enough to move, she began to try to get up. Since she was 69 years old, she was unable to get up, so she started crawling to get to her telephone. She said that she crawled for 5 hours and finally reached the phone and called for help.

She ended up taking an oxygen tank with her wherever she went. She died when she was 71 years old. She was one of the smartest people I ever met about health and could correctly answer just about any problem pertaining to health, EXCEPT HEART PROBLEMS. Unfortunately, she never studied this area and this was her downfall.

After I met her, I learned a lot about all four of the raw drops listed: Raw thyroid, raw thymus, etc. If you feel cold when no one else feels cold, you may have hypothyroidism. I've had this happen to me several times, so I simply get my bottle of raw thyroid out and squirt a dropper full under my tongue, hold it there for 20 seconds, and then swallow it. In rapid time, I no longer feel cold when I shouldn't. You can buy books on hypothyroidism and learn numerous ailments which may be cured or helped by using raw thyroid. I also carry raw thyroid tablets with me when I travel, since I may need them. I also use raw thyroid as well as raw thymus to strengthen my immune system. I sometimes will also use the raw multiple glandular and multiple organ for strengthening my immune system.

GLUTATHIONE

We know that there are many ways that we may increase our health and improve our wellness. One of the surest ways is to increase our glutathione levels. Why should this be great for us? The answer is because each and every disease begins with a decline in our glutathione levels. If you take a look at the many miracle antioxidants which we take, most of the healing effects we receive from them comes from the fact that they raise our glutathione levels. There are many substances which we may take that will raise our glutathione levels. Bilberry extract, grape seed extract, Pycnogenol from pine bark, and tumeric, all improve our glutathione levels. Melatonin, which is great for helping us get to sleep at night, even strengthens dropped production of glutathione peroxidase, which is the principle enzyme which controls free radical damages in our brains.

When we have low glutathione levels, we are much more likely to develop cataracts, cardiovascular diseases, AIDS, Alzheimer's, macular degenerations, Parkinson's, and other aging diseases in general.

In some tests which were done on mice, which had been chosen to develop inflammatory bowel diseases, researchers noticed a great drop in the glutathione level when the mice developed this disease. When they checked this out, they learned that the glutathione levels had dropped a whopping 80%. So the researchers decided to see what would happen if they reversed the glutathione levels upward, so they added N-acetylcysteine to their water. As the glutathione levels increased, the irritable bowel syndrome decreased. So, from these results, we may infer that if we take glutathione each day, we will be much less likely to come down with any disease since our glutathione levels should become very high after a few weeks.

ANTI-CANCER STRATEGIES

In a number of studies, as many as 46% of those cancer patients tested had scurvy, or a total lack of vitamin C. Our immune systems can't function properly without vitamin C. One problem that we develop without vitamin C is our Phagocytic cells (white blood cells that consume cancer cells and other disease-causing organisms) work very poorly or not at all if there is not enough vitamin C in our bodies. When a cancer patient arrives in one of the two clinics hereinafter listed, one of the first things they will do is test you to determine what percentage of phagocytes will gobble up foreign particles such as yeast. This is very low- a normal finding would ordinarily prove that between 40% and 70% of your cells will engulf the yeast. Unfortunately, the results are usually so low you can't believe it. You would probably score as low as a 1 or 2%, which is totally inadequate. One lady who scored this low, took two weeks of therapy and raised her score to 99%, which is extraordinary.

We need lots of vitamin C in our bodies inasmuch as vitamin C is essential for the production of collagen (the sticky substance which holds our arteries together). If we have lots of vitamin C in our bodies, this prevents the spread of cancer throughout our bodies. If you are low in vitamin C, then your immune system is compromised, and will not fight cancer effectively, and our collagen will not withhold penetration by the tumor cells. Vitamin C has been found to induce acoptosis, or programmed cell death, in cancer cells. If you have lots of vitamin C, it is toxic to tumor cells and can prevent metastases, spread of cancer, which causes secondary tumors.

The amount of vitamin C needed by each patient varies between 25 and 150 grams. It would be impossible to take this much vitamin C without developing diarrhea. It would also be impracticable for anyone to take this much vitamin C except intravenously. The labs start patients with 25 grams of vitamin C in an IV, and then perform a test called G6PD to determine if the patient has enough enzymes for his body to withstand much larger amounts of vitamin C without suffering any red blood damage. The amount of vitamin C needed is dependent upon the person's height, weight, body surface and disease process. Those found to have many tumors will need much more vitamin C than someone with only one tumor.

Studies have found that about 80% of the cancer patients have gone through a very stressful period between 6 and 18 months before their cancer diagnosis, and this helps support the theory that they need lots of vitamin C now. The labs have found that by taking 6 nutrients, the patient will need much less vitamin C. The nutrients are bioflavonoid quercetin, lipoic acid, grape seed extract, biotin, niacinamide and vitamin K. (These are all members of the B family.) The amount of vitamin C needed to destroy 50% of the tumor cells in a patient dropped from 700 mg/dl to 120 mg/dl when lipoic acid was added to the vitamin C.

The two laboratories mentioned where you may get excellent treatments are as follows. The Aidan Clinic in Tempe, Arizona, (toll free call to them at 877-585-7684) and also The Immune Institute in Huntington Beach, California (call them toll free at 888-570-1320). The Aidan Clinic has 7 anti-cancer strategies and The Immune Institute has 12 anti-cancer strategies for patients.

If you would like to receive information about cancer on a regular basis, you may do so by becoming a member of the International Association cf Cancer Victors and Friends by sending a $25 check to Mrs. Grace Moore, President of the Northern California Chapter, 5336 Harwood Rd , Dept. 7, San Jose, CA 95124. You will also receive names of people who have beaten cancer who are willing to talk with you and share information as to how they did it. You may telephone her at 408-448-4094.

MORE ABOUT PARKINSON'S

There are some simple steps we may take to protect ourselves from Parkinson's Disease (PD). We've known for several years that people with elevated levels of homocysteine, the amino acid, can cause us to get heart disease, Alzheimer's and other diseases. Scientists weren't certain which came first, the high level of homocysteine, or did the homocysteine rise to a high level because people developed Parkinson's? The studies that have been done showed that high homocysteine levels may lead to Parkinson's Disease (PD).

PD is caused by the progressive degeneration of neurons, or nervous system cells, in the part of the brain which controls voluntary movement. This nerve degeneration causes a shortage of dopamine, the brain hormone or neurotransmitter, which is produced in the brains being studied. A group of laboratory mice was divided into two groups and one group was given a folate deficient diet and the other was given a standard diet, for three months. (Note: Folate deficiency is the primary cause of high homocysteine levels.) The mice on the folate deficient diet developed an eight-fold increase in the plasma concentration of homocysteine compared to the other mice.

The test was carried to a further level when both groups were given the same amounts of MPTP, but the folate deficient mice showed tremendous motor dysfunction after taking this drug. Also, the folate deficient mice lost more that half the neurons in the key brain region, and had lower levels of a dopamine producing enzyme whereas the other group showed no differences in brain chemistry.

Since we know that elevated levels of homocysteiene increases your chances of developing PD, we should all take vitamins B-6, B-12, and folic acid, and should also eat lots of fruit and vegetables. Most doctors will tell you that you should keep your homocysteine level below 12 micromoles per liter. In order to make certain that I get enough B vitamins, I take a capsule with a combination of all the B vitamins each day. I also take B-6 and folic acid every other day, and occasionally I take B-12. I also make it a point to eat fruit and vegetables every day, if at all possible.

If you haven't ever had your homocysteine level tested, you should do so right away. It is a very simple blood test which may be done in any lab or doctor's office. If your level is too high, hopefully you will be able to bring it to a good level using these ideas.

HOW YOU MAY REDUCE YOUR HIGH BLOOD PRESSURE

The first six of these answers is for items to avoid or reduce. The second six of these items are substances you may take to reduce your HBP. Here they are:

- No alcohol
- No smoking (not even second-hand smoking)
- No cola drinks
- No coffee
- No chocolate
- Reduce stress
- Take allicin (included in garlic or can be bought separately)
- Take oleuropin (found in olives and olive oil)
- Calcium Magnesium (take just before bedtime and it will help you sleep)
- Chelation therapy (may help increase your life expectancy)
- Taurine

- CoQ10 (be sure to take L-Carnitine, which improves on the effectiveness of CoQ10.)

SOME ANTI-OXIDANTS YOU MAY TAKE

We know that anti-biotics only kill bacteria, so we may want to take anti-oxidants to kill viruses, and many other parasites.Some anti-oxidants to try, are:

- L-Glutathione
- L-Cysteine
- Zinc Glutonate
- Citrus Bioflavonoids
- Choline
- Inositol
- Beta Carotene

I highly recommend the L-Glutathione and L-Cysteine.

STILL MORE ABOUT PARKINSON'S

CoQ10 apparently slows the progressive deterioration of function for patients provided they are in the early stages of Parkinson's disease. When a number of subjects with Parkinson's took 1,200 mg of the antioxidant CoQ10, they showed a decline in muscle movement and mental function of about 40% less than the placebo group. (Of course, if you are in the late stages of Parkinson's, you should try this also as it may help enough to make you glad you did. It certainly can't hurt to try it.)

L-Glutathione, if taken in large doses, is very beneficial in giving very great relief from the tremors. It should be no problem to take a 500 mg tablet two times a day and see if this helps. If you want really large doses, you should find a medical doctor who can give you injections of L-Glutathione, but if you can't do this, I would try taking two 500 mg tablets per day as some is better than none.

Chapter Twenty

Anthrax

A major part of our news now consists of information as to what is happening in the war which the U.S. has declared against terrorists, and how many people have been exposed to the deadly Anthrax bacteria.

Unfortunately we do not know a lot about Anthrax, but I expect we will soon know a lot about it. During medieval times, Black Bane was the name given to Anthrax as they knew it. This was because of the blackened areas of dead skin of infected persons. The word Anthrax comes from the Greek word "anthrakis", which mean coal.

We know that Anthrax is a disease of sheep, goats, cattle, deer, camels, and others. For some reason, dogs, cats, and rats are very resistant to Anthrax infections. I believe this is possibly because they are able to produce their own vitamin C, in large quantities, and we are totally unable to do so. Maybe our scientists will delve into this to determine the reason why these animals are immune to this terrible disease.

Until recently, we used to record only about 1 case every 10 years in America, and now, during 2001, we have had probably 50 cases up to this date. To my knowledge, only 5 or 6 people have died here with this problem. This would seem to make it only a teeny problem and not something to really do much worrying about. We just have to use our common sense and make sure we don't open our mail and breathe in any Anthrax powder. As Neal Boortz, a great radio announcer, said, he's "more afraid of all the 16 year old children whose parents bought them a car and turned them loose on the highway than he is of the Anthrax." He said he has a much better chance of being killed or injured due to meeting one of these 16 year olds on the highway than he does of being killed or injured from Anthrax.

Probably the largest epidemic of Anthrax took place in Zimbabwe between 1978 and 1980, in which about 10,000 people contracted the disease. This disease is reported to still occur in South America, Africa, and Asia.

No one really knows exactly how much Anthrax it would take to cause us to become infected with Anthrax, but those who claim to know, say it would take at least 10,000 Anthrax spores to contaminate us and send us to the hospital. We would have to breathe this many spores in a short period of time to affect us. The uninterrupted action of the spores would suggest that once we are infected, we stand a good chance of being dead within 36 hours. This is why we need to take action to treat the Anthrax and kill the spores promptly.

Our government claims it is making great strides in our fight against Anthrax, but people are still dying because of exposure to the Anthrax bacteria, or parasites. I have never heard anyone claim that they know that there are no other Anthrax parasites besides bacteria. There could easily be some viruses, or even some other parasites. We do know that bacteria is involved, so we must fight bacteria. If we make preparations to fight other parasites, in addition to bacteria, then we might have a better chance of winning the victory. The government has recommended that we take Cipro to fight the bacteria. This is a drug made by Bayer. In my opinion, we should not just rely on this one drug, plus irradiation which the government plans to treat all of the mail every day. They will probably have to pick and choose. It may also not kill all of the Anthrax, since we do not know exactly how much irradiation will be necessary to do the job. So what else can we do?

COLLOIDAL SILVER

Colloidal silver is great against all types of parasites and they cannot live in even a 5 parts per million silver solution. We know that the silverware we use at home, as well as when we eat out, has silver thereon, and each time we eat with silverware, we consume a small amount of silver and this is good for us to kill parasites in our bodies. Since silver is known to destroy parasites (viruses, bacteria, and all other), it is beneficial to our health to use such tableware. You can buy a CS solution from 5 parts per million to one with 20 parts per million. You may even find it stronger than 20 parts per million.

When I first read that CS was effective against 650 diseases and health problems, I got interested in it and bought some with 5 parts per million. The plastic bottle contained only 4 ounces of CS and set me back $30, although the listed price was $40. I checked other vitamin stores and found one which sold 4 ounces of CS which contained 20 parts per million of silver. I knew that I wanted only 5 parts per million, so I diluted it with 12 ounces of distilled water in a bottle. (Note: Never use silverware to measure CS.) I ended up with 16 ounces of 5% CS solution.

I tested my first bottle of CS with only 5 parts per million of silver and it helped clear up my sore throat. I soon learned that I could safely swallow this amount of CS with no adverse effects. I read where one writer claims we can safely take 10 parts per million, but since I only need 5ppm to do the job, I don't feel like taking 10. In one instance, several years ago, I swallowed what I believe was 20ppm of CS and during the night I woke up and my chest was hurting like I was trying to have a heart attack. Since I firmly believed that there was no way that I was going to have a heart attack, I went on back to sleep, even though I realized I had poisoned myself only slightly, and in the morning I neutralized the CS by taking some activated charcoal. I put a teaspoonful of the black activated charcoal in some water, stirred it and drank it. This did the job and I had no more trouble. I felt great after that. The activated charcoal is great to neutralize over 200 poisons in your body and it is good to take some every month for your health's sake.

I do use 20 ppm to gargle when I have a sore throat, and also to kill parasites in my throat. If I had cancer in my throat or in my mouth, I would be gargling numerous times each day with 20 ppm to attack the cancer until I knew it was gone. Of course, I spit it out each time after I gargled. I remember once I went to my dentist because I was having some pain in my mouth. He made several x-rays and determined that I had some bacteria in my mouth causing the problem. He determined that I was suffering with an abscessed tooth. He gave me a prescription for some penicillin, and made an appointment for me to see a specialist who treats abscessed teeth. I decided to start gargling with 20 ppm of CS, and a little over a week later I received a phone call from the abscess dentist's office I had been referred to. The receptionist asked me if I was suffering unbearable pain, and I told her I didn't have any pain, which was true. She was shocked, but I told her I had been treating my problem with CS. She had never heard of it. I knew that parasites were causing the pain to my abscessed tooth, so I started gargling several times each day with 20 ppm of CS. After only a day or two, all pain left my tooth and mouth. The receptionist cancelled my appointment.

We have always known that it would be possible, but not likely, that biological warfare could be declared against America and that we might have to learn how to protect ourselves. Although we know that we are being attacked by Anthrax now, there are many other types of germ warfare that could be used against us. CS is great because we know that parasites cannot live in even a 5 ppm solution for even one minute. They die instantly, so I recommend that you use 5 ppm so you can consume a few swallows. You may use it on the outside of your body and even in your hair, face, and eyes. I quite often release a drop in each eye and it causes my eyes to feel great because it kills all parasites in my eyes. I know that this helps my eyes and believe that because I use this regularly, I will never have any trouble with glaucoma, cataracts, or any other eye disease. Have you ever felt like there were bugs crawling in your hair? If so, try CS on them. It works. There may be parasites crawling in your hair until you use CS on them. The results are predictable and instantaneous.

We know that Microbial Bio Weapons (MBW) are well suited to terrorist warfare. They don't need large quantities in order to deliver the germs to infect us. Only minute amounts of the germs would be necessary to infect us with Tuberculosis, Smallpox, Plague, and Anthrax. Unfortunately, only a small amount of any or all of these could cause deaths of numerous people in a metropolitan area.

We know that many BW grade microbes may be cultivated by utilizing common commercial equipment, such as that used to make cheese. One expert claims that a major BW arsenal could be produced with less than $10,000 of equipment, in an area such as a small garage. Also, it does not take much scientific training and experience for someone to cultivate the BW in a few weeks or less.

So far, we have been exposed only to Anthrax but some of the other types of BW Microbes that could be used to attack us are Tuberculosis, Smallpox, and the Plague. It wouldn't take many of these to impact a large population. Hopefully, we will not have to face any of these BW Microbes ever. If we do, we should have some idea of something we can use to fight back and to win against all or any of them. The CDC has 8,500 employees and they should have already found a number of defenses we could rely upon. Have you heard of any? I certainly haven't, except for the irradiation and Cipro.

LIVING ESSENTIAL OILS

There are several living essential oils that you can order which may help you in your fight against BWMs. Lavender, Oregano, and Theives are the names of them. It would be a good idea for each member of your family to have a bottle of each of these on hand to use as they may need it. In this way, each family member would carry his or her kits for use as it might be necessary. You may buy the 15 milliliter (ml) bottles

from Living Essential Oils from the Sunshine Team as a distributor
from them by calling 1-888-322-6271. There is no point in paying
retail for these oils, when you can easily tell them you want to be a
distributor. Then the price will be as follows: Lavender $18, Oregano
$21, and Theives $27. Your shipping, handling bill will be computed
on the whole amount of your bill.

Lavender: This is known as the "universal" essential oil
because of its worldwide use in healing. It is highly touted for its great
ability to heal severe burns, cuts, bruises, and skin irritations. It is also
widely known for its ability to almost instantaneously cure headaches,
relieve insomnia, alleviate the symptoms of PMS, and reduce stress.
The fragrance is calming and relaxing, both physically and
emotionally. Most importantly, it kills staphylococcus, the typhoid
bacillus, the diphtheria bacillus, the tuberculosis bacillus, as well as
pneumocossus, hemolytic streptococcus, and numerous other
dangerous pathogenic microorganisms, and it also has strong
anti-venom properties as well. Lavender is a plant, the essential oil of
which is widely used in making perfume, but more importantly, the oil
of lavender has long been known to have powerful disease-fighting
properties. In fact, recent scientific and medical research has proven
that the essential oil of lavender has immune stimulating and
anti-microbia properties that rival, and even surpass many modern
antiseptic chemicals and antibiotic drugs.

Oregano: Sometimes what passes for "Oregano" is actually a
variety of another herb, Thyme. For therapeutic applications, however,
it is extremely important that the extract of genuine oregano be used.
Like extract of Cinnamon Bark, this oil has powerful anti-microbial
properties and has been used widely to combat bacteria, mycobacteria,
fungi, viruses, and other parasites.

Theives: One of the major oils in this formula is an extract of
Cinnamon Bark, which has long been recognized to have powerful
anti-microbial, anti-infectious, anti-bacterial, anti-viral, and
anti-fungal properties.

WHY SHOULD WE USE ESSENTIAL OILS INSTEAD OF HERBS?

Recent research shows that essential oils placed on any part of your body will have an effect on every cell in your body within 21 minutes. This stands in marked contrast to the average of 13 to 23 hours for the therapeutic constituents of dried herbs to reach the cells of the human body after ingestion. Essential oils are extremely concentrated, particularly when they have been derived through distillation, which is the most effective method of extraction. The oils contain virtually all of the plant'' healing nutrients, oxygenating molecules, amino acid precursors, coenzyme A factors, trace minerals, enzymes, vitamins, hormones, and more. Because these essential oils are so highly concentrated, most of them are at least 50 times more therapeutically potent than the herbs or plants from which they are derived. Essential oils are a great choice for the terrorist threats we face as we will be doing our family a favor by ordering for everybody in our family old enough to understand what to do.

EUCALYPTUS OIL

WARNING: This can be toxic if taken internally. Just breathing the oil's fumes will probably knock out infections in your nasal passages, sinuses, bronchial tubes, and lungs without the use of antibiotics or antioxidants.

Dr. David Williams, who is a great doctor, states that he bought a 4 ounce jar of this oil from a health food store. He claims that he put between 8 and 10 drops of Eucalyptus Oil on a small rag every few hours and kept the rag nearby for the next several days. Sleeping with the rag right next to his bed worked wonders for him and allowed him to get much needed rest.

If you should have a cold, flu, or some other discomfort, you might want to try this oil by breathing fumes from drops as Dr. Williams did.

It should help improve your sleep as well as your breathing, and may even knock out some of the infections you are suffering with.

LET'S KEEP THINGS IN PERSPECTIVE

America is in the midst of a full-blown panic over the hand full of deliberate attacks involving Anthrax. But we need to keep things in its proper perspective. Although several hundred have been exposed to this bacteria, only 5 or 6 have died from it. Let's look at some of the latest statistics on the annual leading causes of death in our country.

Heart Diseases	724,859 deaths
Cancers	541,532 deaths
Strokes	158,448 deaths
Obstructive Pulmonary Diseases	112,584 deaths
Pneumonia/Influenza	91,871 deaths
Diabetes	64,751 deaths
Automobile Accidents	47,000 deaths
Suicides	30,575 deaths
Chronic Liver Disease/ Cirrhosis	25,192 deaths
Murders	18,272 deaths
Falls	14,900 deaths
Accidental Poisonings	8,600 deaths
Drownings	4,000 deaths
Killed by Fires	3,700 deaths
Choking on Food	3,300 deaths
Firearm accidents	1,500 deaths
Poisoning by Gases	700 deaths
Surgical Screw-ups	500 deaths
Heatstrokes	30 deaths
Struck by Lightning	15 deaths
Farm Animals	12 deaths
Exploding Tires	10 deaths
Methane Gas	10 deaths
Anthrax	6 deaths

So you see, the number of deaths by Anthrax is really so small that we should not spend any of our time worrying about it. We should just be careful when we open our mail and wash our hands afterwards. The odds are so great against any problems, we should not make a big deal out of it.

Chapter Twenty One

DMSO

Exactly what is DMSO? It is also referred to as Dimethylsulfoxide, which is a great, great drug. As a matter of fact, it is one of the few drugs that I have any use for. I normally avoid drugs completely in the belief that all drugs are poisonous and that drugs do not heal. Fortunately, this is one of the few really good drugs that does seem to heal numerous things. As you probably know, all drugs have side effects, and if there are no side effects, then it is not a drug. DMSO has only one side effect, and this is that it may cause you to promptly develop an oyster taste in your mouth. This is one side effect that I believe we can all live with. The really great thing about this drug is that it is not only safe, but it works to help overcome numerous diseases, as you will see.

USE PHARMACEUTICAL GRADE ONLY

DMSO is a solvent used for cleaning and there are at least two grades of it. The best grade is the pharmaceutical grade as it is pure and has no impurities in it. A gallon of the pure DMSO will cost you about $41, and you can probably buy it from a veterinarian. They use lots of it for the animals in their care which are in pain. If you can't get it from a veterinarian, you may be able to buy it from a health food store. If their best grade comes in dark and light, be sure to buy the light, as this is best. (Note: You will always mix DMSO with distilled water in some combination to take orally, IV, or topically. You will never take it straight.)

Buy some distilled water and mix with DMSO as follows: 70/30. DMSO is 70% of the mixture and distilled water is 30% of the mixture. As an example, pour 7 ounces of DMSO into a plastic container and then pour 3 ounces of distilled water into it. It will get very hot, but don't let this bother you. You may use the combination (70/30) for massaging sprains and other external uses. You'll be quite surprised how far this mixture will go. (You will normally mix it 50/50 for internal use.) Let's say you sprained your left ankle. You would massage the whole left foot and then your ankle and massage about a foot above your ankle. It will take about 15 minutes to dry, so then you may put on a second and third coat of this mixture.

DMSO MAY HELP
IN THESE AREAS

- Sprains
- Stroke (You should mix 50/50 and may swallow a small amount of this mixture plus some orange or other juice.) One lady gave her son a plastic teaspoon of this mixture plus orange juice every fifteen minutes for two hours and then gave him the same amount every 30 minutes for two hours. He regained the use of his arms and legs as well as speech, and had a complete recovery. (Note: If this treatment is given soon after the stroke manifests itself, you may be able to dissolve the clot that caused the stroke.)
- Head injuries (Combine DMSO and fructose diphosphate and have a medical doctor administer this intravenously.) It may help prevent the brain from swelling and causing your death.
- Spinal cord

- Improves circulation (Once DMSO gets into your body, whether given by mouth, IV, or daubed on your skin, it will permeate your body and cross the blood brain barrier, so even if you did take it orally, it can dissolve the clot.)
- Dilates your blood vessels (This causes the carotid artery blood flow to the brain to increase.)
- Increases oxygen
- Intravenous (Thirty minutes after receiving, there is an increase in the flow of cortisone.)
- Alters some of the effects of brain stroke
- If you are already paralyzed, it may help you to regain the use of your limbs.
- If you take L-Dopa and DMSO IV, the DMSO will carry the L-Dopa across the brain barrier into your brain and then the L-Dopa becomes dopamine and turns off that part of the brain that causes a person with Parkinson's to tremble.
- Heart attacks and angina
- Intestinal cystitis
- Bursitis
- Burns
- Arthritis
- Frost bite
- Schizophrenia
- Scleroderma
- Lupus
- Viruses (Flu, Pheumonia)
- Quadriplegics
- Cancer (DMSO + Hematoxylon IV, or a number of drops in distilled water)
- Retinis pigmentosa, macular degeneration and cataracts (only 2 drops in each eye of 50/50 solution: 50%DMSO, 50% distilled water)

- Others (There may be numerous other areas where DMSO will help.) One thing is sure. All claims indicate that it has never hurt anyone whether taken internally (50/50) or for eyes.

In the February 2004, "Second Opinion" of Dr. Robert Jay Rowen, he says: "Knowing that glutathione concentration in the lens is essential for cataract prevention, I thought I would try adding some to the DMSO. Researchers discovered in the early 1900s that eyes deficient in glutathione were more susceptible to cataracts and other eye diseases. I also knew that the sclera of the eye is dependant on vitamin C for good health, and cataracts may begin when vitamin C becomes deficient. So I decided to add vitamin C and glutathione to the formula. I expected the DMSO to carry the nutrients to the lens where they could do their work. And it does seem to work better than the DMSO alone." They claim you need a prescription for this.

You may buy this formulation from Dollar Drug of Santa Rosa (707-575-1313) and the formulation is as follows:

DMSO 6.25%, Vitamin C 1.25%, and Glutathione 1.25%.

Dr. Rowan says "I'm using it myself just for prevention. It stings momentarily and quickly passes. Your eyes will love you for it."

I recommend that you obtain several good books about DMSO and learn all you can from them. Here are several of them: Politics in Healing by Daniel Haley; DMSO, The Pain Killer by Dr. Stanley Jacob and Robert Herschler; DMSO, Nature's Healer by Dr. Morton Walker and he also wrote Coping With Cancer. You may order these last two books from Freelance Communications, 484 High Ridge Rd., Dept. 7, Stanford, CT 06904.

WARNING: Never put DMSO into glass, always use plastic.

Chapter Twenty Two

The Ultimate Healer

When you learned you had cancer, you found this hard to believe, but finally you realized that you are not indestructible and you accept this as a fact- YOU DO HAVE CANCER AND MUST DO SOMETHING ABOUT IT.

Regardless of what you decided to do about it, you finally reach the conclusion that the treatment didn't work and YOU ARE NOW DYING OF CANCER. You don't know how much time you have and neither does your doctor; he only says that you are dying of cancer and you may die anytime, or you could even live 30-60 more days. At any rate, he says that he is not God and doesn't know exactly how much time you have left.

You finally realize that you don't know any other treatments than the operation you had, the chemotherapy you took after the operation, and the radiation you took after the chemotherapy have failed. (Your doctor also claims he doesn't know any other treatments that he would recommend.) You went through all these treatments, and it has now been over a year since you started this series of treatments. The doctor told you that your cancer was in remission, when he made the first examination after the operation was complete, but now says that the cancer has returned. Now you believe that your cancer never left you because the cause of cancer was never eliminated and only the symptoms were removed when you had your operation. You have even learned that you have secondary cancer from the treatments. Why didn't the doctor tell you that you could get secondary cancer from the chemotherapy and radiation treatments?

ONLY GOD CAN HEAL YOU

When all else has failed, and you learn from a very reliable source that you are dying, what else can you do to get healed? Your only hope now is to turn to the ultimate healer. If you believe in Jesus, you know that He can heal you no matter what the circumstances are or the problem is. Sometimes, such as now, you realize that He is the ultimate hope, and if this doesn't work, then you must know that you are on your way to the cemetery. (Note: If you are Jewish, you must try what several of my Jewish friends have done. They tried praying to Jesus for the desired results, and sure enough He came through for them, and they realized He is for real. Two such friends did this and are now very devout Christians. PRAISE THE LORD!)

You have been a Christian for many years and have been going to church, but you have been donating only $1 each Sunday, even though you know from the Bible that as a Christian, you are required to donate a tithe, which is at least 10% of your total income, plus offerings. In Malachi 3:8-11, in the King James Version of the Bible, it says: "Will a man rob God? Yet ye have robbed me. But ye say, wherein have we robbed thee? In tithes and offerings. Ye are cursed with a curse: for ye have robbed me, even this whole nation. Bring ye all the tithes into the storehouse, that there may be meat in mine house, and prove me now herewith, saith the Lord of hosts, if I will not open the windows of heaven, and pour you out a blessing, that there shall not be room enough to receive it."

Another thing you must realize is that you can't go to the Lord and ask for his help and blessings and tell him that you are holding ill feelings, grudges, hatred, or other bad feelings towards anyone and expect Him to hear your prayers and grant your requests. It simply is not going to happen, unless you come to Him with clean hands.

So what should you do now? Since you are holding a grudge or ill feelings against several people, you must now forgive them and write each of them a letter telling them that you forgive them, and ask that they forgive you. You must in fact forgive them, because you can't fool Jesus. He will know if you are only pretending, so make sure you really and truly do forgive each of these people, and write and mail the letters telling them this. Your very existence may depend on this. Remember, this is your LAST CHANCE!

Since you've been stealing the Lord's money for all these years, you should now make a supreme effort to make it up entirely, plus pay extra. Instead of giving a tithe, you should now give 15% or 20% of your total income and make a promise to Jesus that you will do this from now on until you have more than repaid the money you stole from God. Remember, He trusted you with all of the money you received and only asked for 10% plus offerings in return. You decided you could spend and use this money better than Jesus could, so you stole it from Him.

Now that you set both of the above corrections into place, you may do one or more things to get healed. You can find a spirit-filled Christian and get him or her to pray for your healing to take place, and then you must accept the healing for it to be effective. If you go back to your doctor for more of his treatments, you have not accepted, nor do you believe healing by God took place.

ANOTHER IDEA FOR HEALING

Since you are now a "King's Kid" with all the rights as a Christian, you can take authority over your disease and start praying for Jesus to heal you. You might read one of the many passages on healing in the Bible and say the passage each day for a while, or you might say this to your body: "The healing power of Jesus is flowing all through my body. Every cell in my body is being bathed in the healing power of

Jesus, and is being healed. All diseases in my body are being healed and all infirmities are being cured. No disease or infirmity can prosper in my body against the great healing power of Jesus. Thank you so much Jesus for healing my cancer and infirmities. YOU'RE SO GREAT."

I suggest that you say this healing prayer at least 7 times per day. Seven is a good number and Jesus likes this number. I recommend that you use it every day. And, keep on paying the tithe, plus extras, and offerings each week when you go to church, and read your Bible from cover to cover. Please don't forget to pray every day also.

LORRAINE DAY, M.D.

Now I want to tell you a short story about a medical doctor who got cancer and what she did about it. She starts out by stating that if you have cancer, you are one of the lucky ones. She claims this because she says this because when you get well, you will have it made from now on, or words to this effect. You will be well and will know how to stay well and free of cancer. She says she taught thousands of people the wrong information because she didn't know any better.

BREAST CANCER

She was informed that she had breast cancer and this caused her to have the lump removed, but she refused to have a mastectomy. She changed her diet because she knew that 1/3 of all people who have cancer may get rid of it by changing their diets. Nine months later, she learned that diet was not enough in her case, as her tumor returned. This time she had an incision biopsy. She really gave it her best effort to lick her cancer by taking at least 40 different treatments to see if they would work and cure her cancer. Unfortunately, she got no better. As a matter of fact, her tumor grew from a marble size to grapefruit size, and was even sticking out of her chest. Her tumor was now the size of a softball and was extremely painful. She refused chemotherapy and radiation, was bedridden, and was sent home to die. She spent lots of time searching medical literature and finally came up with 10 rules which you may now follow to get your cancer well. These rules are totally natural and have no side effects. Don't worry about losing weight while you are following these rules because the foods which make you gain weight helps feed the cancer, what it needs to do you in. You can gain the weight back after you have overcome the cancer and prove this by valid medical tests. Dr. Day states that the number one cause of death is anger. Here are ten rules (laws of life) given by Dr. Day which she followed and got well:

- Stop doing the things which caused cancer. (Note by author: As an example, if you have colon cancer, stop eating all beef. If you have cancer in other parts of your body, stop eating all animal foods, such as fish, chicken, beef, etc.) Resort to proper nutrition, and eat as close to natural as possible. Her only exception was to eat lots of brown rice. The best idea of all is don't eat any meats.
- Exercise. You may reduce the chance of breast cancer by as much as two-thirds with 4 hours a week of exercise. Walking will do if you can't do other exercises.
- Drink lots of good water. Your body is 75% water and needs lots of water. Drink lots of fresh natural juices each day freshly squeezed by you or someone in your home. If you have any room left, then drink 4 or 5 glasses of some good spring water or other good water.
- Get lots of sunlight. Go out early in the morning and gradually work up to one hour of sunshine per day. Make sure that you don't get burned.
- Sugar has to go as it paralyzes the immune system.
- Get lots of fresh air. If you are in a hospital, you breathe lots of stale air.
- Get the proper amount of rest each day.
- Learn how to handle your stress, and, if possible, do whatever is necessary to eliminate your stress.

- You must have an attitude of gratitude to God. Remember, healing comes from God and not by drugs or by man. God healed Dr. Day of her cancer or she would be dead now. She did what was necessary to be healed.
- Be benevolent. Selfishness is a great killer. You brought nothing into this world when you came into it, and it is certain that you will take nothing out.

Cancer doesn't scare me anymore. We know that chemotherapy is poison and that it not only poisons you, it also causes secondary cancer. The same is true of radiation. It will cause secondary cancer also. Both of them will destroy your immune system, and you NEED YOUR IMMUNE SYSTEM as this is what will make you well. You got cancer because you had a weak immune system, so what does your doctor do? He decides to destroy what is left of your immune system even though what you really need is to strengthen your immune system. You have to wonder if all doctors are crazy.

Chemotherapy and radiation never does destroy all of the cancer cells. Radiation causes the cancer cells to spread (metastasize).

Dr. Day says it took 3 months to get rid of her tumors.

Chapter Twenty Three

How to Add Ten to Fifteen Years or More to Your Life

If you are young, you may add more than 10 to 15 years to your life by adopting these ideas hereinafter set forth. If you are seventy, you still may be able to add ten or more years to your life.

We know from reading medical information that numerous doctors believe that we will die a natural death when our immune systems are unable to handle the toxins and poisons which have accumulated in our bodies, so let's see if we can't reduce the amount of poisons and toxins which are in our bodies. The least this will do is to make us feel better and stay healthier. We will have less colds, flu, pneumonia and many other diseases. It may even make us well from some disease which we are having trouble defeating.

1. GET RID OF YOUR AMALGAM FILLINGS NOW!

First, you must get rid of all of your nickel silver amalgam fillings as they are poisoning you twenty-four hours per day. If you read the book "It's All In Your Head," you will discover that numerous diseases are caused by the poison from fillings. When you chew gum or eat, this causes an excessive amount of toxins and poisons to circulate throughout your body and it must be stopped promptly.

Go to your dentist and get him or her to remove all of these fillings and replace them with composite fillings which have no silver or other harmful metals. Get the gold removed from your mouth also as it is unnatural and causes some degree of toxins in your mouth and body.

2. ELIMINATE ALL SODIUM FLOURIDE FROM YOUR CONSUMPTION

We all know that sodium flouride is the second deadliest poison known to man, and only arsenic is more poisonous, and therefore we must start buying and drinking distilled or spring water. I recommend the spring water three weeks in a row and then distilled water for one week. The distilled water may help to act as a cleanser. Carry a bottle of water with you everywhere you go and you will drink much less of the bad water being forced upon us. Above all, do not use toothpaste with flouride in it, as it has 1,000 times more flouride in it than is in your water.

Flouride destroys collagen in your arteries and may cause you to develop an aneurysm, which can be fatal. Calcium flouride is the way the Lord makes flouride and this is not poisonous. Sodium flouride is man-made and is very poisonous. We know that sodium flouride may cause us to develop cancer and other ailments.

3. CLEANSE YOURSELF INTERNALLY TO REMOVE TOXINS

If you will purchase the four items Dr. Schulze sells for your health, they will go a long way towards improving your health now and in the future. The four items are as follows: Intestinal Cleanser #1, Intestinal Cleanser #2, Echinacea Plus, and SuperFood. You will start taking #1 first with your main meal at night by swallowing one of these capsules with some water. If you don't get three good bowel movements the next day, you then take two capsules the next night, and, if you still don't have 3 good bowel movements, you will add one more cleansing capsule each day until you get 3 good bowel movements. I know I only needed one of these capsules to start with, and then after over a year, I started taking two capsules each night with good results. You will be surprised how many toxins and poisons will be eliminated from your body in this way each day.

After you have taken this Intestinal Cleanser #1 for a week and had good results, you will then take Intestinal Cleanser #2 with some fruit juice up to five times in one day. This will clean out the feces which were missed by #1. You will continue to take IC #1, even though you are taking IC #2, each day.

By taking Echinacea Plus and also SuperFood, you will strengthen your immune system and improve your health. If you also take the juice fast for 30 days and also adopt the vegan vegetable diet, this also helps very much.

4. ENJOY A GOOD JUICE FAST TWICE A YEAR

Drink all the fresh squeezed orange juice you want (or other fresh juice of your choice) for five days, or longer, and fast to further cleanse your body of toxins and poisons. This will do wonders for your health. Do this in addition to numbers 1, 2 and 3 previously listed.

5. CLEANSE YOUR LIVER AND KIDNEYS

You may buy a liver cleanser from Dr. Schulze and also a kidney cleanser from him. He recommends that you take each of them every three months. I have taken both of them and it is not bad at all. When you take the kidney cleanse, it may help you to overcome your incontinence.

You may order these from Dr. Schulze by dialing 1-800-HERB-DOC. Ask what their special for the month is, as they usually have at least one special every month. They also have some package deals which may result in a savings to you.

6. GET EXERCISE AND SUNSHINE EACH DAY

Be sure to get plenty of exercise and sunshine each day, if possible. When you get into the sunshine, the rays of the sun will go into your body through your eyes and help you stay healthy and strong. Do not look directly into the sun as this is not necessary to get these benefits. I suggest that you get at least 20 minutes of sunshine, if possible.

7. AVOID TAKING DRUGS IF POSSIBLE

If you are taking illegal drugs to get high, you may wind up in the morgue at a young age or at least way before you would have died under normal circumstances. This is like taking a pistol with only one bullet in its chambers and playing Russian Roulette. You may win once or twice, but why play a game which may destroy you?

If you take drugs prescribed by your doctor, do you know all of the side effects of each of these drugs? Sometimes you may find that a side effect is that "THIS DRUG MAY KILL YOU." We know that over 100,000 people die each year from iatragenic drugs, which means drugs prescribed by a medical doctor. Ask your doctor what the side effects of the drug being prescribed are, and if he doesn't know, BEWARE. I would be sure to find out what the side effects are as it's your body which will suffer from the side effects, and you're just another patient to the doctor. He won't worry about the consequences you suffer from taking the drug he prescribed. If it kills you, he will just say, "We can't win them all."

8. BUY YOUR DRUGS FROM CANADA TO SAVE MONEY

If you must continue to buy drugs and take them for health reasons, you may be able to save a considerable amount of money by purchasing them from Canada.

If you have a prescription, you may telephone 1-888-800-0328 to a drug store in Canada to make your purchase. You will be required to mail your prescription to them after you have determined that the savings are substantial. An example of a substantial savings is as follows: One person determined that the cost of having his prescription filled here in the U.S. would cost $145, but he learned he could buy the same drug in Canada for $90, a $55 savings.

One possible reason why the drugs are so much cheaper in Canada than they are in the U.S. is because we have so many suit-minded lawyers and individuals in the U.S. who will sue for almost any reason. We recently learned that lawsuits have been filed against McDonalds and other hamburger outlets, claiming that the plaintiffs became fat from eating their hamburgers, french fries and other items. What could be more ridiculous than this? If McDonalds had refused to sell hamburgers, french fries and other items to the plaintiff, he would have sued and claimed he was being discriminated against, so he seems to be saying to them that they will lose either way. I can't believe such a lawsuit will prevail as it is totally frivolous and the court should throw the plaintiff and his attorney out of court and make them pay all expenses of their opponent.

If you purchase over the counter drugs, you must make certain you know all of the side effects as these drugs may make you sick or even kill you. I was just reading where a physician says, "Toss your Acetaminophen, for your liver's sake." It seems that people were buying over-the-counter such drugs as Excederin, Tylenol, and Anacin-3 and that 30% of all liver cases or unexplained liver failure at hospitals are directly caused by the Acetaminophen doctors prescribe. Of course, these 3 drugs listed contain Acetaminophen, so toss them.

9. DON'T SMOKE AND AVOID SECOND-HAND SMOKE

We all know that smoking may kill you and certainly won't improve your health. My sister smoked herself to death and so can you! It took her three packs a day for 40 years for her to do it, but she died because she couldn't breathe. I'm sure you'll agree that this is a horrible way to die. I know I smoked for 14 years and have to admit that this is absolutely DUMB. It's plain stupid to do this to your body. I learned that if you really want to quit smoking, you may buy some black licorice and each time you feel you must have a cigarette, you simply eat a piece of black licorice. I have read that more people claim that black licorice helped them more than anything else to quit smoking. I certainly hope that you will do this if you are a smoker who is determined to stop this ridiculous habit.

You should avoid second-hand smoke as this is still smoking and may cause bodily harm to you eventually.

10. ELIMINATE OR REDUCE THE SWEETS IN YOUR DIET

Cancer needs glucose to survive and sugar and other sweets is just what they need. I suggest that you reduce or eliminate all sugar, honey and other sweeteners from your diet. It will make it tough for cancer to ever establish a colony in your colon or other part of your body. If you strengthen your immune system as set forth in this book, this will also help to eliminate cancer from your body as well as keep it out permanently. It may also eliminate polyps.

One bad thing which may happen to you from eating too much sweets, is you may find that you are having dizzy spells, and there may be times when your balance is gone and you can hardly walk. You may be disoriented also, so I hope you will heed this warning.

11. REDUCE OR ELIMINATE ALCOHOL FROM YOUR DIET

Although a little alcohol in your diet may be good for you, if you cannot control your drinking so that you only drink a small amount of wine or beer two or three times per week, you would be better off if you did not drink at all. If you do drink, I suggest only one glass of wine or two beers when you drink. It may actually be good for your health to do this, but you must not drink every day or even close as you may lose control over your drinking and become a confirmed alcoholic.

12. ELIMINATE ALUMINUM FROM YOUR DIET

We know now that aluminum is bad for your health. You may end up with Alzheimer's from too much aluminum. Avoid drinking soft drinks or beer from cans since you will get aluminum in your body each time you do so. Also, throw away all aluminum cookware as this really loads you down with aluminum every time you eat. Buy stainless steel instead as this is safe. Avoid taking Tums and all other things which have aluminum in them.

Remember, sodium flouride causes your body to retain aluminum and it will ultimately go to your brain and you may end up with Alzheimer's Disease. I recently read that if you will take 600 mg of Alpha Lipoic Acid each day, this will stop Alzheimer's in its tracks.

13. AVOID TAKING ASPIRIN TO THIN YOUR BLOOD

Dr. Bill Douglas, a great doctor, said "if you have a headache caused by an aspirin deficiency, then you should take aspirin." He also said, "The much promoted physician's health study proving that taking aspirin regularly will prevent heart attacks didn't use just aspirin, but aspirin plus magnesium in the form of Bufferin. Research years ago proved that magnesium protects the heart." GREAT IDEA- Take Bromelain instead of aspirin.

14. ELIMINATE STRESS FROM YOUR LIFE

We know that stress enters your life when you become distressed. Stress can cause you to lose sleep, become highly nervous, and even keep you from thinking right. It may even cause you to lose control of your car and have a horrible crash. There is one thing we know it will do. It will shorten your life if you don't get rid of the stress, so I recommend that you do whatever is reasonably necessary to eliminate it if it lasts for days or weeks.

One thing you may do to eliminate stress is "don't hold a grudge." You must forgive the person causing stress and make up, if possible. If you caused a problem with another which caused the stress, you may apologize and ask for forgiveness. If you have made reasonable efforts to overcome your stress but failed, one thing you can do is to "give it to God." We know He can handle it and can make you well. Sometimes this is the only way. He can make a way when there seems to be no way. In 1 Peter 5:6-7, the Bible says, "Cast all your anxiety on Him because He cares for you."

15. EDTA CHELATION THERAPY WITH SUPPOSITORIES

Some people have tried oral Chelation Therapy, but in my opinion, this is not as effective as suppositories. EDTA is largely destroyed during digestion, greatly diminishing its effect. IV Chelation Therapy is great but the cost is prohibitive and you may need 30 treatments, which would cost over $3,000. It normally takes at least 3 hours per treatment, which is also a drawback.

New research indicates that removing heavy metals through chelation can treat and/or prevent many serious diseases such as pancreatitis, gout, rheumatoid and osteoarthritis, chronic fatigue, irritable bowel syndrome, Alzheimer's disease, cancer and multiple sclerosis. Each suppository is taken just before bedtime, and delivers 750 mg of EDTA. Three of these is equal to the one gram delivered by IV treatment.

The name of it is Detoxamin, and it costs $299 for 30 of them from World Health Products. Telephone 877-656-4553. If you will buy a box of 30 of these (or more, if needed) and take the Liver Cleanse every 3 months, you will improve your health and may add years to your life. By taking Intestinal Cleanser #1 and #2, you may also remove excess metals from your body.

16. YOUR IMMUNE SYSTEM

Your first line of defense when a disease, virus or other sickness comes your way is your immune system. What is your immune system? It consists of the following: tonsils and adenoids, thymus, spleen, bone marrow, appendix, emotional dialogue, lymphatic field (white blood cells) and Peyer's patches.

Some of us have parents who inherited very strong immune systems, and we inherited very strong immune systems from them. If we happen to be born of parents who have very weak immune systems, we will probably also have very weak immune systems. In addition, if we live very long lives, we probably have immune systems which are getting weaker and weaker each year. We all have cancer, but if it has not manifested itself because our immune systems have been strong enough to keep it under control, we are very fortunate. Should our immune systems decrease in strength until they cross the line of resistance for our cancer, we will then realize we have cancer.

17. REBUILD YOUR IMMUNE SYSTEM

If this happens, it would be logical to rebuild our immune systems. It would be better still if we would strengthen our immune systems each and every year to keep them strong. Why wait until we have cancer to start doing this? How can we strengthen and rebuild our immune systems? It is possible to have a medical doctor measure our immune system's strength so that we know how strong or weak it is. Normally we would score between 45% and 65% of the maximum, but sometimes a person will have an immune system that is so weak that the person will only score a 10%. How can you rebuild your immune system in a hurry? You may find a medical doctor who, after you have taken three or four of these treatments, probably over a period of several weeks. may help you to score about a 90%. You would then have a very strong immune system.

In October, I took an intravenous treatment of one liter of ascorbic acid and this December I took an intravenous treatment of one liter of H_2O_2 (Hydrogen Peroxide), to protect me from parasites and diseases. I took this treatment because it may help my arthritis and also because it will kill parasites in my body. Sure enough, it did help my arthritis. I also take 5,000 mg of Omega 3 for my arthritis each day and this also helps.

Another excellent treatment which you should take to strengthen your immune system is the Echinacea Plus offered for sale by Dr. Schulze. You should keep several bottles of this on hand and take it at least one month a year to rebuild your immune system.

I have read the names of a number of people who had cancer and discovered an excellent treatment which ultimately cured their cancer. Sometimes a person who learns of this will take the same treatment and their cancer is not cured by it. I believe that it depends upon the strength of their immune systems. If you have been taking chemotherapy or receiving radiation treatments for your cancer, you may have weakened or even destroyed your immune system. Now that you have nothing to fight with, how can you hope to defeat cancer or any other disease with no immune system?

Of course, you may take multiple glandular or multiple organ drops to strengthen your immune system. Raw thymus and raw thyroid may also help. I keep raw thyroid on hand and if I ever realize I am cold when no one else is, then I take a dropper full and this does the trick.

You may also take 1,000 mg tablets of ascorbic acid each day. You may start with 500 mg tablets if you wish, but I prefer the 1,000 mg tablets. You should aim to reach a goal of 10,000 mg per day of ascorbic acid. You may start by taking one tablet after each meal and then one at bedtime. If you are finally taking the 1000 mg tablets, this is 4,000 mg per day. You may wish to gradually increase to 2,000 mg first thing in the morning and 2,000 mg after each meal and 2,000 mg at bedtime. If you happen to have arthritis, you may be surprised how much this will help you. Nearly 100% of those who have arthritis are VERY deficient in vitamin C and even border on having scurvy; over 40% probably do have scurvy. If you start taking vitamin C as previously recommended, and your urine doesn't become very yellow, you badly need this vitamin C. Vitamin C will help build and repair collagen, an essential part of your cartilage.

18. HOMOCYSTEINE

If you have an increased blood level of homocysteine, an amino acid, you may have poor heart health. It is best if it is below 12 micromoles per liter. A high homocysteine level may cause cognitive difficulties, moodiness, deep vein thrombosis, heart and brain problems, intermittent claudication (leg pain), poor circulation, bone loss, and numerous cardiovascular difficulties. If you drink 8 or more cups of coffee per day or consume lots of alcohol, you will probably raise your homocysteine level. Men have more risk than women and seniors have the greatest risk inasmuch as they probably have deficiencies of B-12, B-6 and folic acid. This especially causes a decrease in cognitive function. They need to flush out the arteries and may do so if they take the amino acids L-Lysine and L-Proline. You may buy L-Lysine and L-Proline 500 mg in one capsule and take one each day. They may also flush the arteries with oral or intravenous chelation, which would have to be given to you by a medical doctor. If you flush out the arteries, you may reverse the effects of aging. Poor cardiovascular function may cause age related senility and cause a diminished flow of blood which leads to diminished sexual function.

You may normalize your homocysteine by taking the following B vitamins: 800 mcg of folic acid, 800 mcg of vitamin B-12, and 100 mg of vitamin B-6. By taking this daily for 6 weeks, 100 men with hyperhomocysteinemia reduced their plasma homocysteine levels by 49.8%. See Journal of Nutrition, 1994, 124, 1927-1983.

In healthy individuals, homocysteine levels are low. You may have your medical doctor run a blood test to determine your level **of homocysteine.**

19. AVOID ASPERTAME

In some of the early tests on aspertame, it caused microscopic holes and tumors in the brains of experimental mice and caused epileptic seizures and heart attacks in monkeys. It also was converted into formaldehyde.

Aspertame is now included in over 5,000 processed foods. You should read the labels of all such foods carefully as you must avoid consuming any product containing aspertame- YOUR LIFE DEPENDS ON IT. Avoid Nutrasweet and Equal as well and stop drinking diet drinks. Michael J. Fox, a former Hollywood actor, developed Parkinson's and when he was asked how he got it, he replied, "I drank 10 Diet Pepsi's every day."

Over 144 million Americans eat and drink low calorie, sugar free products such as artificially sweetened soda pop and deserts. Ten percent of aspertame is methanol, a deadly poison also found in wood alcohol.

Methanol becomes more dangerous when heated above 86 degrees Fahrenheit before being consumed. If food or drinks containing aspertame are left out in the sun or heated when being prepared, this causes the methanol to break down into formaldehyde and formic acid in our bodies. This is very toxic to you in this form. Full strength formaldehyde is embalming fluid. Nothing can live in its presence. It inhibits oxygen metabolism. Your heart muscle and brain both need lots of oxygen. Formaldehyde is very toxic to us and may cause eye damage and birth defects.

Phenylalanine and aspertic acid constitute 90% of aspertame and are neurotoxic. Components of aspertame when ingested go straight to our brains. This causes faulty balance, seizures, headaches and mental confusion.

Over 450,000 people in our country are victims of sudden death. Many high school and college athletes suddenly die. An American Airlines pilot was drinking a diet drink and suddenly fell over dead. The other pilot landed the plane safely. President Bush fainted and claimed it was due to a pretzel he ate (which contained aspertame.)

A lady named Kathy believed she was dying because she was having blackouts. Ten doctors could not determine the cause and then a friend talked her into not consuming any aspertame product and she never had any further health problems. Another friend of hers drank diet drinks to keep her weight down and also suffered blackouts. She was recently found dead on the floor of her house.

STOP DRINKING CARBONATED DRINKS

A study of 500 athletes determined that drinking even one carbonated drink per day increased the fracture rate of bones from 200% to 500%. (Note by author: I suspect that drinking carbonated drinks regularly may cause our hip bones to fracture, causing great problems and pain to us.) Coke was claimed to be the worst offender. Carbonated beverages may also cause you to have heart problems, so to stay healthy, you must stop consuming them.

Drinking carbonated drinks will block the ability of your body to absorb calcium as well as magnesium. These are essential to your health.

For additional information on aspertame, read Aspertame Disease: An Ignored Epidemic, by H.J. Roberts, M.D.

MORE INFORMATION

BOOKS THAT WILL CHANGE YOUR LIFE:

BEHOLD I SHOW YOU A MYSTERY

Softback, 124 p. $9.95
ISBN- 0-9601416-5-0

END TIMES HANDBOOK- TAKE A LOOK AT THE
DANGEROUS EVENTS JUST AHEAD, BE READY

TABLE OF CONTENTS:

1. The Mystery
2. The Order of Events
3. When Will the Rapture Happen?
4. Judgements and Prophecies
5. The Antichrist System
6. Antichrist- The Man & His Reign
7. The False Prophet
8. The Apostate Church
9. The True Church
10. The World During the Tribulation
11. Endure to the End
12. Be Prepared

HOW TO MAKE YOUR OWN WILL
(With tear-out Will Forms)

Softback, 64 p, ...$14.99
ISBN- 0-901416-6-9

THIS WILL HAS IT ALL! It provides for the division of property, a personal representative to execute your will, even a Trust for minor heirs.

All you have to do is fill in the names, and other pertinent information according to the simple instructions. Sample paragraphs are even included to cover special situations.

This impressive, air-tight document has been prepared by J. Eugene Wilson, J.D. author of HOW TO FIGHT THE IRS- AND WIN! Dr. Wilson is a well known Atlanta attorney with over 54 years experience.

He has done careful research and guarantees the Will to be valid in all States except Louisiana.

"...I found this book to be very helpful and instructive in preparing one's Will without fuss and furor, and with legality.

...it is well worth the price to make sure it will be your decision and not the State's as to where your estate will go. I recommend it most highly."

Doris Benbow, President
ATLANTA WRITERS CLUB

HOW TO FIGHT THE IRS- AND WIN!

Hardback, 368 p,..............$24.95   ISBN- 0-9601416-4-2
Softback, 368 p, ...$19.95   ISBN- 0-9601416-3-4

Highlights of this amazing book:

- Pitfalls to avoid at audit
- How to handle a discourteous agent
- What to do if your answer will incriminate you
- Dangers of conferences with the Appellate Division
- A secret that can keep you out of prison
- An idea that settles cases
- How to receive a fair trial
- How to avoid IRS seizure of your records
- How to obtain info with the Privacy & F.O.I.A. Act
- Records and proof required
- What to do about a summons
- How to prepare a petition for filing in Tax Court
- How to use interrogatories to discover the Commissioner's evidence
- Other discovery methods explained
- When you may file suit in the "Small Tax Court"
- How to prepare a brief
- How to avoid preparing a brief
- Avoiding an increase in your deficiency

ABOUT THE AUTHOR: J. Eugene Wilson, Juris Doctor has practiced law for over 54 years, and specializes in income tax cases. He is the author of "How To Fight the IRS- and Win!" and "How To Make Your Own Will."

"… the book is written for laymen and is packed with useful information. If you are facing an audit of your federal tax returns, this book by an Atlanta attorney could be helpful." – *The Atlanta Journal & Constitution*

HOW TO FIGHT
THE IRS- AND WIN. II

Softback, 212p ....$19.95   ISBN- 0-9601416-7-7

This amazing book will show you...

HOW TO SUE AN IRS AGENT & MAKE HIM PAY YOU.
Learn how to sue an IRS agent or nearly any other government official
who violates your Constitutional rights. You win and he pays out of
his own pocket! Largest judgement to date against an IRS official-
$200,000.

HOW TO SUCCESSFULLY OPPOSE AN AD VALOREM TAX
INCREASE ON YOUR HOME

HOW TO TOTALLY AVOID WITHHOLDING LEGALLY.
Who is and who isn't subject to withholding laws. Must you use the
W-4 form?

HOW TO HAVE CHARGES OF TAX EVASION, TAX FRAUD,
FAILURE TO FILE & MUCH MORE THROWN RIGHT OUT OF
COURT. Discover the little known loophole which won the case for a
tax rebel and has been winning ever since for those in the know.

KEY CASES WHERE TAXPAYERS WON SIGNIFICANT
VICTORIES AND CONCESSION. Here's just a sample:

We find it intolerable that one Constitutional right should have to
be surrendered in order to assert another. (U.S. Supreme Court)

The claim and exercise of a Constitutional right cannot be
converted into a crime. (U.S. District Court)

Once challenged, the burden of proof of jurisdiction rests with the
IRS. (U.S. Supreme Court)

HOW TO PROVE THE IRS HAS NO JURISDICTION. An actual
appeal from the U.S. District Court, which successfully challenged the

jurisdiction of IRS is reproduced. The author explains step-by-step how to use this pleading to win your own case.

STATUS OF OUR CURRENCY. Use this information to your advantage on contracts and on any lawsuit which concerns money (even criminal charges)

Information and pleadings which are both practical and helpful on money, audits, U.S. Tax Court, and lots of other areas which will enable you to deal successfully with the obstacle course we call the IRS.

Mr. Wilson is one of the special attorneys authorized to present cases to the U.S. Supreme Court.

THE SANHEDRIN PAPERS
(including the gospel of Judas)

Written by Charles A. Schafer
$19.95

This is the story of Q. Scholars in the Bible field have generally agreed that the Gospel authors based their books on a previously written work known as Q. This is basically a story of Christ, told through the eyes of those that lived with him and knew him. It is a biographical novel which- to a point- follows closely the general knowledge about Christ; then it goes on to specific items of interest which make this book an outstanding contribution to the religious literature of our day. This is perhaps the real truth about Christ and the way it really happened. You'll really enjoy reading this book.

SHADOW OF DEATH

Written by Frieda Turner
$14.95

Learn the shocking truth about our prison system. In 4 minutes Tommy Callahan will be executed... but he is innocent!! Tommy missed execution by four minutes in 1952, and his sentence was commuted to life imprisonment. During the 20 years that followed, Tommy was beaten, starved, shot, escaped and recaptured. In 1957, he was transferred to the Rock Quarry Prison at Buford- Georgia's punishment camp where inmates broke their legs with sledge hammers and cut their heel tendons with razor blades to protest the brutality and inhumane punishment. A true story, written in easy to read, simple language. Shadow of Death relates Tommy'' traumatic 31 years of a living hell while confined in various Georgia and North Carolina prisons. He finally won his release at age 45. An outstanding book.

TAX TARGET: WASHINGTON

Written by Gary Allen
Softback..........$3.95

This book shows you how billions upon billions of your tax dollars are wasted by Washington every year. It proves that the federal budget could be trimmed $100 billion a year, without hurting a single important program. It reveals the only way to halt sky-rocketing taxes and spending. The part you must play in bringing the monstrous federal bureaucracy under control. (With a special introduction by Howard Jarvis- Proposition 13 sponsor in California.)

INDEX

A

A, Vitamin 97, 155, 168
Auto Immune Deficiency Syndrome (AIDS) 23, 51, 59, 99, 202, 281
Alcohol 76, 99-102, 155, 285, 311, 316
Allicin 112, 170, 285
Aluminum 110, 163, 171, 176, 311-2
Alzheimer's Disease 56, 59, 110, 163, 211-2, 281, 284, 311-3
American Cancer Society 29
Amino Acid(s) 53, 97, 185, 205, 209, 273, 284, 293, 315-6
  Homocysteine 284-5, 315-6
  L- Arginine 185-6
Anthrax 287-91, 294-5
Antibiotics 31, 89, 110, 114, 136, 270, 293
Anti-depressant(s) 75-6, 93
Antioxidant(s) 212, 281, 286, 293
Appendix 250, 313
Apple Cider Vinegar (ACV) 158-60
Arthritis 21, 46, 116, 153, 164, 180, 183, 269, 298, 314-5
Ascorbic Acid 214-5
Asparagus 149, -51
Aspertame 316-8
Aspirin 60, 95, 98, 153, 312
Asthma 107-8, 158, 161, 234

B

B-6, Vitamin 168, 316
B-12, Vitamin 97, 211, 316
Bacteria 35, 60, 88-9, 98, 100-8, 113-5, 180, 201, 286-92, 294
Bad breath 20, 172, 177
Blood 29-31, 46, 52-7, 60, 67-8, 74-7, 86-7, 96-9, 118, 123-4, 130-1, 135, 137, 151, 154-5, 159-62, 175, 180, 182-6, 193, 201-2, 205, 207-10, 212, 214-5, 270, 275, 277, 279, 282-5, 298, 312-6

Red Cells 97-99, 182
 White Cells 46, 60, 97, 201, 282, 313
Blood Pressure 56, 75, 123, 154-5, 161, 183, 185-6, 210, 215, 285
Bone Marrow 124, 129, 313
Bone Marrow Transplant(s) 31-2
Breast Cancer 31, 33, 51, 94, 134

C

C, Vitamin 204, 282-3, 287, 299, 315
Calcium 18, 67-8, 155, 180, 285, 307
Calcium Flouride 307
Cancer(s) 19-36, 40, 44-46, 49-52, 59, 101-2, 110-1, 116-24, 129, 133-38, 141, 143, 147-52, 155, 161-4, 169-71, 174-7, 179, 181-7, 190, 192-9, 201-8, 215, 249-50, 256, 269-84, 290, 298-307, 311, 313-7
 Breast Cancer 31, 33, 51, 94, 134
 Colon Cancer 32, 45, 51-2, 152, 202, 278-9, 304
 Lung Cancer 21, 148-9, 182
 Prostate Cancer 33, 51, 275-7
 Thyroid Cancer 144
Carrot (juice) 24, 58, 132, 164
Cayenne 24, 60, 61, 73-6, 112, 125-6, 167, 183-5
Chemotherapy 21, 27, 30-4, 45, 117, 124, 127, 129, 131, 133-4, 137-9, 148, 205, 278-80, 300-3, 305, 315-6
Cherries 155, 164
Chocolate 25, 108, 285
Chorionic Gonadotropin (CG) 30-1
Crohn's Disease 45, 47, 154
Cigarette(s) 25, 64, 89,310
 Smoking 21, 25, 64, 76, 285, 310-1
Coffee 43, 132, 285, 316
Cold(s) 64, 103-15, 141, 143, 172, 201, 214-5, 234, 27, 293, 306
Cold Sheet Treatment 19, 24-5, 59-60, 144
Colitis 45, 47, 154, 216
Collagen 282-3, 307, 315

Colloidal Silver (CS) 53, 165, 289-91
Colon Cancer 32, 45, 51-2, 152, 202, 278-9, 304
Constipation 37, 39, 41-5, 51-6, 79, 82, 86-7, 101, 114, 161, 167, 173, 176
CoQ10 (Vitamin Q) 204-14, 273, 286
Cystitis 161, 298

D

D, Vitamin 97, 152, 155, 168, 278-9
Dementia 46, 56, 101, 247, 255
Depression 38, 46, 57, 83, 101, 121, 181, 274
Diabetes 21, 101, 116, 161-3, 186, 215, 269, 294
Diarrhea 161, 172, 283
Digestion 29, 46, 96-7, 101, 160, 313

E

E, Vitamin 97, 211
Echinacea Plus 36, 45, 49, 90, 108, 111, 115, 135, 143-4, 167, 307-8, 314
Ellagimax 32-3
Emphysema 161
Epileptic Seizures 161
Erectile Dysfunction 73-6
Exercise 42, 44, 65, 82, 121, 126, 162, 174, 304, 308-9

F

Fat 57, 84, 97, 210, 310
Fava Beans 155
Fertility 56, 71
Fever 60-1, 107-8, 111, 113, 172, 234, 251, 253, 257
Fish Oil 151-55
Flu Shot(s) 109-10, 156-7
Folic Acid 205, 208, 211, 285, 316
Foods

Apple Cider Vinegar (ACV) 158-60
Asparagus 149, -51
Carrot (juice) 24, 58, 132, 164
Cayenne 24, 60, 61, 73-6, 112, 125-6, 167, 183-5
Cherries 155, 164
Chocolate 25, 108, 285
Coffee 43, 132, 285, 316
Fava Beans 155
Fish Oil 151-55
Garlic 40, 46, 61, 69, 94. 104, 112-5, 126-7, 157, 160-1, 169-70, 285
Ginger 25, 46, 60, 112, 215
Juice 24, 36, 47-9, 58, 89, 95, 97, 108, 111-3, 132, 140, 143-4, 164, 175-7, 297, 308
Sugar 96, 146, 174, 227, 275, 304, 311
Tea 25, 35-6, 60-1, 75, 84-5, 88, 112-3, 126, 146, 161
Fruit 47, 113, 164-5, 171-2, 176, 285, 308

G
Garlic 40, 46, 61, 69, 94, 104, 112-5, 126-7, 157, 160-1, 169-70, 285
Ginger 25, 46, 60, 112, 215
Gout 164, 270, 313

H
Hair (loss) 33-4, 137, 168
Headache(s) 28, 58, 82-3, 153, 164-5, 167, 172, 177-8, 181, 269,-70, 292, 312
Heart Attack 99, 154, 184, 208, 213, 289
Heart Disease(s) 101, 116, 141, 164, 212, 284, 294
Homocysteine 284-5, 315-6

I
Immune System 60, 101, 106-7, 110-1, 114, 129, 131, 157, 186, 205, 207, 271-83, 304-8, 311-5
Impotency 63, 68, 70-3

Incurables Program 19, 66, 116, 125-7, 134-5, 140, 142
Indium 181-3
Infection(s) 52, 56, 74, 87-90, 100, 103-14, 136, 161, 175, 232, 235, 269-70, 287, 293-4
Infertility 56, 63, 68, 70-3, 88
Influenza (flu) 103-6, 109-15, 130, 141, 156-7, 173, 201, 215, 293-4, 298, 306
Intestinal Cleanser(s) 36, 49, 307-8, 313
Intestinal Detoxification Program 46
Irritable Bowel Syndrome 35, 47, 282, 313
Iron 97, 99

J
Jaundice 99-102
Juice 24, 36, 47-9, 58, 89, 95, 97, 108, 111-3, 132, 140, 143-4, 164, 175-7, 297, 308

K
K, Vitamin 97, 283

L
L- Arginine 185-6
L- Carnitine 309-11, 273, 286
L- Proline 316
Liver Kampo 214-5
Lou Gehrig's Disease 144
Lung Cancer 21, 148-9, 182
Lupus 154, 201, 298

M
Magnesium 18, 155, 285, 312
Melanoma 179, 181, 274
Microbes 29-31, 291
Migraine(s) 153, 165-6, 177-8, 270
Minerals

Indium 181-3
Iron 97, 99
Magnesium 18, 155, 285, 312
Multiple Sclerosis 154, 313

N
Nausea 34, 82-3, 181, 161
Nitric Oxide 185
Nitrogen 185

O
Oleuropin 285
Oxygen 97, 162, 180, 185, 275, 277, 281, 298

P
Pain 32-3, 37, 41, 53-4, 82, 86-8, 95, 98, 103, 120, 130, 136, 144, 153, 164-7, 181, 228-9, 275-6, 290, 296, 299, 315
Pancreas 55, 86, 131, 179
Parasite(s) 16, 40, 46, 48, 98, 170, 200-2, 272-3, 286, 288-92, 314
Parkinson's Disease 144, 155, 182, 211-5, 282, 284, 286, 298
Pelvic Inflammatory Disease (PID) 88-9
Peyer's Patches 313
Pneumonia 173, 201, 215, 294, 298, 306
Premenstrual Syndrome (PMS) 56, 80-5
Prostate Cancer 33, 51, 275-7
Psoriasis 154
Puberty 37, 76, 78-80

Q
Q, Vitamin (CoQ10) 204-14, 273, 286

R
Radiation 27, 30, 117, 134, 148-9, 195, 205-6, 280, 300-5, 315
Red Blood Cells 97-99, 182

Rife 269-73

S

Salt Water Treatment 170-8

Smoking 21, 25, 64, 76, 285, 310-1

  Cigarette(s) 25, 64, 89,310

Sodium Flouride 307, 312

Spleen 129, 253, 313

Stress 42, 72, 82, 117, 121, 285, 292, 304, 312

Stroke 99, 101, 154, 164, 280, 297-8

Sugar 96, 146, 174, 227, 275, 304, 311

SuperFood 36, 45, 49, 66, 80, 107-8, 113, 125-6, 133, 135, 144, 167, 307-8

Symptoms

  Constipation 37, 39, 41-5, 51-6, 79, 82, 86-7, 101, 114, 161, 167, 173, 176

  Fever 60-1, 107-8, 111, 113, 172, 234, 251, 253, 257

  Headache(s) 28, 58, 82-3, 153, 164-5, 167, 172, 177-8, 181, 269,-70, 292, 312

  Impotency 63, 68, 70-3

  Infection(s) 52, 56, 74, 87-90, 100, 103-14, 136, 161, 175, 232, 235, 269-70, 287, 293-4

  Nausea 34, 82-3, 181, 161

  Pain 32-3, 37, 41, 53-4, 82, 86-8, 95, 98, 103, 120, 130, 136, 144, 153, 164-7, 181, 228-9, 275-6, 290, 296, 299, 315

  Stress 42, 72, 82, 117, 121, 285, 292, 304, 312

T

Thyroid Cancer 144

Treatments

  Cold Sheet Treatment 19, 24-5, 59-60, 144

  Echinacea Plus 36, 45, 49, 90, 108, 111, 115, 135, 143-4, 167, 307-8, 314

  Exercise 42, 44, 65, 82, 121, 126, 162, 174, 304, 308-9

  Intestinal Cleanser(s) 36, 49, 307-8, 313

Intestinal Detoxification Program 46

Salt Water Treatment 170-8

SuperFood 36, 45, 49, 66, 80, 107-8, 113, 125-6, 133, 135, 144, 167, 307-8

Tuberculosis 161, 217, 233, 249-50, 252, 256, 291-2

Tumor(s) 24, 29-31, 46, 52, 117-8, 137, 144, 149, 182, 185, 202, 206, 215, 276, 283, 303

V

Vegetables 18, 24, 40, 113, 129, 172, 285, 308

Virus 60, 88, 98, 100, 104-8, 113, 115, 156-7, 271-2, 313

Vitamins

A, Vitamin 97, 155, 168

B-6, Vitamin 168, 316

B-12, Vitamin 97, 211, 316

C, Vitamin 204, 282-3, 287, 299, 315

D, Vitamin 97, 152, 155, 168, 278-9

E, Vitamin 97, 211

Folic Acid 205, 208, 211, 285, 316

K, Vitamin 97, 283

Q, Vitamin (CoQ10) 204-14, 273, 286

W

White Blood Cells 46, 60, 97, 201, 282, 313